The Gateway to 10,000 Illnesses

Bio Craniopathy and a Trailblazing Discovery Revealed

by

Robert Boyd, D.O.

Foreword and Edited by
Tom Tessereau

ISBN 978-1506-907-25-3 PBK
ISBN 978-1937-520-34-2 EBK

Published by First Edition Design Publishing

July 2023

www.firsteditiondesignpublishing.com

To all those nameless souls who have dared to challenge.

Acknowledgements

In compiling this book, I am deeply indebted to all those practitioners who have long since seen "the cause behind the cause" and who have selflessly and enthusiastically continued to support me in my endeavours, often in challenging circumstances. To "The Team" especially go my boundless appreciation for being there for me and helping make it all worthwhile – Dr Norm Price, Dr James Augustine, Dr Carl Blomencamp, Dr Cruse C Howe (and his late father, Dr Cruse J Howe), Armando Jarrin, CBC, Dr Judy Peterman and, not least, the late Dr David Driscoll. And many others.

I would specially like to thank Tom Tessereau, CBC, for his unstinting contributions of time, energy and resources to help in establishing the ***Bio Craniopathic*** mission and laying the foundation of the new discipline of ***Bio Craniopathy***. My thanks also go to his staff, without whose time and support none of it would have been possible.

Finally on the scene to help me refine ideas came Kieran Burke, CBC, who has been a most wonderful support in more ways than one.

To Linda Montgomery again go my thanks for her superb artistic work in helping me explain some of the principles involved. Any confusion remaining can be entirely laid at my door.

Disclaimer

This book has been published to provide the physician, and the reader, with additional information with which to make informed judgments about health protocols which may be of benefit to themselves or others.

The understandings and experiences described are not intended to replace any advice from one's chosen doctor, and are not being suggested as specific medical treatments. At all times it is recommended that the reader seek appropriate medical advice for any medical condition, be it for oneself or any loved one.

Contents

Foreword

Greetings and welcome to the world of **Bio Craniopathy**. This book will redefine everything you currently know about healthcare and how the human body functions. This is one of those rare finds that will change your life because the principles within are indeed ground breaking and paradigm shifting.

As you read this book, I wonder if you will notice that you are in the presence of greatness. What will you see, what will you need to hear, what will you need to feel within yourself to help you to understand that you are witnessing, within this book, medical history in the making?

I would like to share with you what I will call the story of two Michaels. Of course, North American readers will know that Michael Jordan is considered by many to be the greatest basketball player in the history of the game, even by some to be the greatest player of any sport. And yet his high school coach in tenth grade cut him from the team, because the coach did not have the ability to do what I am inviting you to do, which is to read between the lines, hear between the notes, and get a sense of something that is subtle and not so obvious, which in this case was that the coach had before him one of the greatest athletes of all time and he didn't even notice.

The second Michael is, ... perhaps you heard about this in the news in 2010. A middle-class family living in Buffalo, New York had a painting hanging in their home for generations. And in 1972 one of the kids hit it with a tennis ball and it fell behind the couch and it stayed there until recently when it was discovered that it was actually a very rare painting by

Michelangelo, estimated at approximately 300 million dollars in value.

Isn't it interesting they didn't know they were in the presence of a masterpiece... of something great? Perhaps it is about timing, so maybe it is too early for some to know, and to experience, to feel, to hear, to see and appreciate the masterpiece that the author, Robert Boyd, has created. Many will realize this treatise marks the beginning of a new era in medicine because it reveals the art, the science, and the philosophy, behind **Bio Craniopathy**, a new discipline, a new understanding, a new day in healthcare.

These writings are the culmination of the unique research carried out by the author, a United Kingdom based Osteopathic physician, regarded worldwide as a pre-eminent researcher and lecturer. I admit that I didn't understand initially what people were saying about Robert being another Einstein, or Da Vinci. I must say that I didn't at first notice that I was in the presence of greatness, but have come to know him as not only a brilliant mind, a seeker, a kind and gentle man, he also possesses an unsurpassed humility.

My name is Tom Tessereau, Certified **Bio Craniopath** and Executive Director of the Bio Cranial Institute International. I have been studying Complementary and Alternative Medicine for more than 35 years and have been a full-time practitioner and teacher for more than 20. And yet, perhaps like you, until I met the author of this book, I was still looking for the key that unlocks the hidden power of the body to heal itself.

It gives me a great deal of satisfaction and honor to present to you the following findings of my mentor and friend, and in the end, a great help to each and every one of us, Robert Boyd,

D.O. and ***The Gateway to 10,000 Illnesses*** - *Bio Craniopathy and a Trailblazing Discovery Revealed.*

~Tom Tessereau

Preamble

There are now a number of cranial groups arising from the premise that there is movement of, and between, the bones of the head. The content of this book is intended to give the reader an overview of the understandings of one of these. They are at the core of a new school and profession called ***Bio Craniopathy***.

Bio Craniopathy began its journey as far back as the late 1970's and early 1980's and was the result of my research into the potential health benefits of the little understood involuntary movement of cranial, and other, structures.

These findings and conclusions were first described and announced to the professional community in my first book, *An Introduction to Bio Cranial Therapy*, published in 1988. The understandings later became known as the *Bio Cranial System (BCS)*. Further additions to these principles and their practical application have now resulted in the establishment of ***Bio Craniopathy*** as a discipline in its own right.

Bio Craniopathy differs from all other cranial groups in a number of important ways, particularly in the analysis of the significance of the moving mechanism in relation to most illnesses and disorders, irrespective of their nature and how and where the symptoms appear in the body.

It also suggests a new status required for the disposition of the cranial bones, in total, if there is to be full functioning of the body's physiological systems. This is a *completely new* concept which I believe all of us must aim for and requires a defined skill to facilitate the cranial bones to assume *that very specific status* one with the other.

Contrary to many cranial understandings, ***Bio Craniopathy*** predicates that the philosophy underpinning it is not merely an aside, relevant only to a limited number of disorders, but is relevant to almost all.

~Robert Boyd, DO (UK)

Preface

Healing, particularly in the Western world, has been highjacked.

There is a tsunami of exhortations telling us that, for our health's sake, we must ensure that we take this or that medication if we suffer from, or want to avoid suffering from, this or that disease. The marketing gurus have fine-tuned their techniques and, not least, have cleverly exploited the *fear* scenario. "If you don't continue to take your medication, your cholesterol will go sky high and you will risk having a stroke…." Or some such thing and one of many examples I have seen over the years.

One of the effects of this kind of marketing has been the creation of a physiological *dependency* on the chemical trade as a necessary requisite to their wellbeing. It has been highly successful for the promoters and it has equally been disempowering for a great number of people.

Perhaps even worse has been the creation of a widespread *dependency*, not only on the chemicals themselves, but of a parallel *intellectual dependency* in many cases, based on *fear*, and on a belief that the normal mechanisms of the body are no longer alone capable of sustaining the life processes. These subliminal messages become entrenched in the subconscious, and so, mission accomplished.

The Orwellian idea of *control* is established to the point of unquestioning *acceptance* by many of us, in the absence of any obvious alternative, that our destiny in the all important area of personal health is *dependent* for its delivery on a range of external sources, not all of which have altruistic motivation. Or results. An empire of providers has evolved to service that dependency.

This is not to insist that there are not circumstances when medication, for example, is necessary, even vital. Nor is it to deny that surgery has its place in health provision, although even then at a much-reduced level from current practice. The vast majority of disorders, however, including injuries, ought to be amenable to conservative approaches for resolution with little, or no, input other than from those forces already contained within the organism.

The answer to *control* and *dependency* must surely be *freedom* and *knowledge*. This book attempts to provide a new understanding, which is itself a step on the road to that objective. But it is also about a *mechanism*, almost unknown in the world of healthcare, and the *freedom* or otherwise for that mechanism to operate, and which, when compromised, will provide the *main basis* for health breakdown on every level. It follows that, if the very *existence* of that mechanism is known, its role understood and its failures addressed, then many things previously thought not possible, become possible.

And we almost all are compromised from birth. Herein may you find answers you are looking for.

~Robert Boyd, DO (UK)

Introduction

Faith is taking the first step even when you don't see the whole staircase.

Martin Luther King, Jnr

The proposition that the head – the cranium – has something to do with health and healing is not new.

The proposition, however, that the cranial mechanism is ***the primary source*** of most dysfunction probably is new and is the subject of this book.

Cranial mechanism? Yes, exactly that. In these pages we will be considering a living, moving and vibrant phenomenon in which motion of the bones of the head is central to practically every area of our health, and its opposite – disorder. The mechanism I refer to is entirely absent from mainstream medical knowledge or, indeed, interest. It follows, therefore, that any suggestion of such a heresy will risk attracting derision and ridicule from the keepers of the entrenched schools of thought.

But then that's the history of medicine.

What follows, however, is an attempt to explain why this missing Big Player is so important and what the mechanisms involved are. And do. Not least, in what areas of illness and disorder the cranial dimension is relevant. Never fear, the descriptions are not dressed up in the language of gobbledegook medicine and are intended to be readily understood. Indeed, these words are particularly directed to the butchers, bakers and candlestick makers of this world to help their understanding and make informed choices about their health and that of their loved ones.

But it is also directed to the health professionals in a wide number of fields, including conventional medicine and dentistry, and including those in such areas as osteopathy, chiropractic, acupuncture, natural medicine, naturopathy and so on, in the hope that the message will perhaps give cause for reflection.

It may come as a surprise to some that the idea of the head - the skull - having *something* to do with health goes back a long way. For example, there is extensive evidence of the widespread practice known as *trepanation* having been carried out by early civilisations in many areas of the world from as early as Neolithic times (circa. 4000 – 2000 BC) in France. It appeared in many civilisations over the years in the Americas, Europe and Asia. The practice involved the boring of holes in the skull of living beings and is believed by present day scholars to have been part of early primitive medical procedures, as well as religious ones such as the releasing of evil spirits.

Medicine certainly was primitive in ancient times but, one assumes, and crude as it was, there must have been some perceived "benefit" for the patient, even if we can only guess at what the survival rate might have been.

The practice of applying manipulative techniques to the bones of the head is a much more recent addition to the sum of knowledge and a number of schools have evolved during the past 80 years or so. Cranial manipulation, too, has had a controversial passage within the professions concerned and continues to this day. My own introduction to cranial work came about by way of the osteopathic school – known as Cranial Osteopathy - and this insight was sufficient to convince me that the cranial dimension had not yet been fully explored and that it held the key to untold potential in the healing arts. The problem, as I saw it, was that nowhere could I find the answers I was looking for.

The simple reason was that they didn't exist.

The understandings arising from my own research in the 1970's and 80's resulted in an entirely new appreciation of the role of the cranium. As you may imagine, these conclusions, by implication, were challenging to a number of prevailing views, including those already in the cranial field.

They also suggested that our knowledge of the role of structures such as the spine was incomplete.

From all of this was born a new approach to which I gave the name, *Bio Cranial Therapy (BCT)*, and which later became known as the *Bio Cranial System (BCS)*. This, in turn, has now become ***Bio Craniopathy*** which has, as its core basis, a philosophical understanding based on the existence of a moving mechanism first suggested by the American Osteopath, Dr. William Garner Sutherland. There is nothing new about that, insofar as much existing cranial work is based on Sutherland's original discovery.

What is new, however, is that the ideas underpinning ***Bio Craniopathy*** predicate a specific objective, anatomically and physiologically, which *must* be achieved for *all* of us. That objective *is completely new and original* in the field of cranial work, and while it is not intended to immerse the reader in the technicalities of that objective, the understandings in what follows will provide a clear overview both of the significance and potential of the cranial mechanism.

Both the theory and practical work embodied in ***Bio Craniopathy*** are unique and far removed from previous cranial practices. Within these pages are contained a broad panorama of some new ideas.

Part 1

Function

Creating a new theory is not like destroying an old barn and erecting a skyscraper in its place. It is rather like climbing a mountain, gaining new and wider views, discovering unexpected connections between our starting points and its rich environment.

But the point from which we started out still exists and can be seen, although it appears smaller and forms a tiny part of our broad view gained by the mastery of the obstacles on our adventurous way up.

Albert Einstein

Chapter 1

Dys-*Function*

Wealth is the product of man's capacity to think.
Ayn Rand

Is your heart ticking over? Well, it has to be, of course, otherwise you wouldn't be reading this. But, *how well* is it ticking over? And that's another question. What I mean is, on the Richter scale of how well you are functioning (1-10), is it ticking over at, say, 4.2 of what it *should* be (10.0), or *could* be? Or maybe 6.8? Or even 9.2? Now, that would be something.

But you don't know, do you?

What am I talking about here? The answer is simply *function*. How well are your bits and pieces *functioning*? How well is your liver *functioning*? Your kidneys? Your thyroid? Your pancreas? Your right knee? Your left eye? And so on. Nowhere in the field of medicine does anyone know the answers to these questions, even though a plethora of tests are made to check areas such as levels of this, that and the other. But none of these will give an overall assessment of the *total* extent to which a system, or organ, is functioning.

In fact, few people even know that these are *the* questions.

Most believe that, having gone through a series of often very sophisticated medical checks and tests, they are determining how well they are *functioning.* And they will obviously be getting *some* information, perhaps about the blood Ph level, about thyroid function, about cholesterol level, about cardiac performance and so on. But, are they receiving any information about their *total* functioning state?

Everything is connected. Everything is inter-dependent and nowhere is there a means of checking the *totality* of that "connectiveness". Which is *function.* The approach that we have settled for is a fragmented one in which our focus is directed to the parts – the kidney, the knee, the lung, the sciatica, etc – rather than the whole. Not surprising, when our cultural approach to healthcare is based largely on the philosophy of *chasing the symptoms.*

Yet, these are questions at the most basic level of our existence. At what is effectively the crudest level of measurement, we largely, though not exclusively, resort to *measurement by symptoms.* We mostly only think we are ill, or dysfunctioning, when we have symptoms. We then only *act* when symptoms arise and, even then, sometimes with reluctance.

We almost all accept that this is a normal and rational approach to measuring, if that's the right word, our health and/or fitness status. If a knee goes pop on the football field then there are symptoms and we know that the knee (and associated structures) has to be investigated and addressed accordingly. Note, I said the knee. Not the pancreas; not the elbow; not the duodenum. We react to the symptoms – the knee.

If you are an athlete your thoughts might turn to your particular sport. You do all the right things. You train hard.

You follow the right nutritional rules. But, if only you could get rid of that nagging, and recurring, ankle problem you know you could get that extra lift, that bit more pace, you know would make all the difference.

Or, if you could conquer that nasty shoulder problem, your serve would be immensely improved. In fact, in no time you would be ready for one of the tennis Grand Slams? What do I hear? Oh, so the shoulder injury occurred five years ago, that time you helped move the sofa into the other room? And it's an injury you have to live with, you've been told by the best? Well, you know what? The best, like all of us, only know what they know. Which means they don't know what they don't know.

Let's define the word "function". On the face of it we tend to think of the word as relating to voluntary activity; that is, how well and efficiently we go about doing ordinary, everyday things. But if we have an injury, say a fracture, then we are not moving too well. We are dys-*functioning.*

Even if we have vague aches and pains, we know we are not functioning at the best level. Nor, if we happen to be a migraine sufferer, are our concentration and decision-making processes at the top of their game. We are not functioning very well *for the duration of the migraines.* But, so what, we'll be back to full throttle tomorrow when it's all gone. Or, will we? Why do the migraines keep coming back?

Then there are those other areas that we don't think of so much as belonging to the category of *function.* It could have been a lifelong problem but it has necessitated a constant reliance on *Cascara sagrada*, or some such laxative medicine, for the constipation you remember going back to childhood. Or, it might have been the all-too-often need to resort to medication for that pesky recurring heart flutter that seems to arise for no apparent reason. These are areas that we don't think of too much as belonging to *function.* They are activities that we do not *consciously* think of as having to be done by us.

They are part of our *involuntary* function.

So is what our liver does (or does not do), without our being aware of it. And our kidneys. And even down to those billions of little cells, beavering away, striving their mightiest to do all those myriad things they were designed to do. And we don't know a fraction of what those are. We are humbled.

But help is at hand, at least to a degree. When we become *knowingly* dysfunctional, which is to say usually when we become aware of *symptoms,* we find that in many cases the body has the ability to heal itself. And by *heal,* I mean ameliorate or clear the symptoms, for - and this is important - most of us assume that, *in the absence of identifiable symptoms,* all is well. However, we will come to that one later.

Admittedly, we all want rid of the symptoms super fast and will turn to various remedies, sometimes any remedies, to obtain relief. But all the while the final resolution process will involve the body's *innate healing processes,* with or without outside intervention.

The surgical procedures will still finally draw on the gift we are all endowed with, that of harnessing the healing mechanisms within, just as those same mechanisms will heal a cut finger. In our minds, increasingly targeted by the vested interests, media and others and their PR machines, we have largely lost sight of, and even confidence in, the simple message expressed in the concept of:

Vis medicatrix naturae **- the healing power of nature.**

We too often lose sight of that simple proposition and attribute the healing processes entirely to external elements. Some typical comments from patients might be as follows:

Sarah: "It was the cider vinegar that cured my arthritis".
Me: (Shhh, *to myself*): "No doubt it helped, but it would have been useless *without the healing power from within".*

John: "I tried everything and it was the Yoga that finally cured my hamstring problem".
Me: (*to myself again*. I'm no fool. I know when to shut up): "Sure it helped to open up to the healing flow from within. It facilitated *the release of the healing power from within*".

You see, the body *does not want* to be dysfunctional.

The body *was not designed* to be dysfunctional.

Even more so, the body is *forever* striving for equilibrium. It never stops, *even in the presence of the most profound disorder or dysfunction*. Now isn't that something? Even when someone is really, really ill, or dysfunctional, that healing stream, that inner intelligence, is striving with might and mane to bring about organization. Which is health.

There are some basic principles, basic truths, that we seem to be increasingly losing sight of and we need to revisit these, almost elementary, concepts in the quest for rational answers.

The guiding principle most of us use to determine how well, or otherwise, we are doing is to acknowledge whether or not there are symptoms present. It's a pretty simplistic formula we use, such as:

"Do I have a pain?"

"Is that a lump I see developing there?"

"What's that blotch on my skin?"

"Why do I keep falling over?"

By implication and, let's face it, an inner hope and persuasion, sometimes driven by fear, we believe all is well, unless there are very definitive symptoms such as those listed above. All of which is very natural and understandable. We want to *believe* all is well and what other yardstick is there to point to the contrary except, perhaps, some of the tests on offer which are routine practice.

By *symptoms,* the general belief is that there is some very definitive departure from what we would regard as *normal,* something that should either resolve by itself or, something for which professional help needs to be sought. The red flag is up. But, the reality is that

none of us knows what "normal" is.

None of us knows what 10.0 on the Richter scale is. You see, none of us has ever been there. From birth. All we know is what is *normal for each of us.*

And that can be, functionally speaking, a long way away from the potential we are capable of.

Let me ask a few questions. Would any of these apply to you, or those within your family or circle:

The impatient ones? Maybe even to the point of having a short fuse?

The shy ones? Maybe blushed easily as a child?

The ones who run out of steam easily, mentally and/or physically?

The regular hay fever sufferers every Spring?

Those who can't stand loud noises?

Perhaps they (or you) prefer putting the weight more on one leg than the other when standing?

Those who screw up the mouth to one side more than the other when talking or laughing?

In fact, have you ever noticed some of the non-laughs of some of the high-profile personalities on your screens? The forced attempt but not quite making it?

But then you wouldn't consider these *real* symptoms, would you? They are not like a pain in your tummy, are they? And yet, I'm sure you would agree they are, what shall we say - *abnormalities*?

Certainly, they are not *disabling* abnormalities. Some of them are almost subliminal in our consciousness; perhaps little more than nuisance value.

Yet they are evidences of departure from what we think of as normal, or balance, and as such, are indicators of a departure from normal *function*. Which brings to mind the truth of the old maxim that I learned as a young man:

"The absence of symptoms is no indication of the presence of health"

When I first heard that one I had no more than a hazy idea of its significance. Healthcare, in the western world at least, is mostly symptom driven, in spite of the marginal, peripheral and sometimes questionable, tests increasingly being introduced. There is little, or no, evidence of any understanding of the mechanisms behind our *functionality* which has to be at the very core of so much of Mankind's dys-*functionality* – illness, disorders, injury.

Functionality is at the very core of the commentaries in this book. It is relevant to what we do and, to a significant extent, who we are. It is the level at which we perform in the turbulent seas of life, about the level at which we exist. It is the measure of our efficiency in our daily tasks. It is about the intrinsic measure of our ability to reduce, or avoid, our exposure to illness, trauma and other assaults on our equilibrium.

It is the central theme of the ***Bio Craniopathy***.

Chapter 2.

The Life Force and Movement

If I have seen further it is by standing on ye shoulders of Giants.
Sir Isaac Newton

In the previous chapter I made reference to the word *function,* and its derivatives, a word which is nothing more than a sensible word for *physiology.*

Physiology itself is, of course, the one half of the Castor and Pollux of medicine - anatomy and physiology. Anatomy is the framework we are provided with and is specifically designed to facilitate all of the physiological processes. Which are? Well, just about everything.

As I twiddle my thumbs, that's function. As my skin sheds its dead matter, that's function. As my fingers write these words, that's function. And as the thought processes which tell my fingers intelligently (most of the time) which keys on my computer to press, well that's function too. There's much co-ordination in all this. And, there's a lot of "intelligence" in all of it too.

The notion of an *intelligence,* a self-regulating, self-healing mechanism, which is the inheritance of us all, required, if possible, that some attempt be made to put it on a scientific footing. One of the early entrants into this area was Walter B. Cannon, M.D., Sc.D., Professor Emeritus of Physiology at Harvard Medical School, who showed, for example, how the body maintains a relatively constant state of salt and water content, of sugar, of acid-alkaline balance, and how it maintains a relatively constant temperature.

Cannon coined the word:

HOMEOSTASIS

to describe the self-regulating ability to adjust the body's level of function *according to its needs*. This confirmed, on a scientific level, what we observe subconsciously on a daily basis, namely, that the principle of *homeostasis* carries with it the concept that the organism not only *requires* certain parameters within which to function, but also has the *ability* to adjust within, *according to its needs.* Cannon's own definition was:

Homeostasis: A homeostatic system is an open system that maintains its structure and functions by means of a multiplicity of dynamic equilibriums rigorously controlled by interdependent regulatory mechanisms. (1933).

By extension, it then begs the question: how does it do it? The body *knows* what it needs to do to function - and to survive! We take it for granted. As sentient beings we don't consciously need to think about it, or try to control it. Let's, for a moment, take a philosophical stroll down the lane of some of the ideas which have relevance to this discussion.

As a boy I recall developing an interest in two closely linked ideas. One was referred to as the *Life Force* and the other as the Vitalistic principle, or *Vitalism*. Incidentally, these concepts apply to all organic matter – the animal and vegetable kingdoms. But let's not get too complicated and let's just consider these in the context of our species, Homo Sapiens. Incidentally, how did our species ever manage to acquire that name – sapiens (wise)?

The two concepts were closely linked, of course. After all, putting it in a negative context, how could there not be a *Vitalistic* outcome from a *Life Force* presence within each and every one of us? If we go back a bit, however, the definition of *Vitalism*, even the very existence of the concept, has exercised the minds of philosophers, biologists, physiologists and others for centuries. And from this, there came to be probably two major opposing camps in the discussion.

In the red corner were the mechanistic biologists, and in the blue corner the advocates of the Vitalistic school. At this time, the Vitalistic school has been on the defensive for some considerable time. There is an obvious difficulty in "proving" the basic principles which underpin the concepts surrounding *Vitalism*. We can't measure it – at least not yet. As against that, others argue, "Why should we ***have to prove*** what is the blindingly obvious?"

My initial exposure to the concepts embracing *Vitalism* came early in my professional career. Let me quote you from one of my first lesson materials:

*All systems of natural healing......., are founded essentially upon one basic principle: that the human organism possesses an inherent urge to protect, regulate, adjust and heal itself. This phenomenon has been observed from the earliest times, and to explain it, many learned men have advanced the theory that a vital force ('vital': **concerned with organic life**, and 'force': **strength** or **intense effort**), permeating the whole organism, was responsible. This vital force has been variously named –*

'Life Force', by the French physiologist, *Claude Bernard,* the *'Dynamis'* by the founder of the homoeopathic school, *Dr Samuel Hahnemann* and the *'Elan Vital'* by the French philosopher, *Henri Bergson.* Bergsonian thinking is often referred to as Vitalism.

I want you to note particularly two definitions:

Firstly, that of ***vital***: - defined as *"concerned with organic life"*, and then the word: ***force***: - defined as *"strength"* or *"intense effort".*

I'll return to these definitions presently.

It was Aristotle who posited the idea that the primary distinction between mechanism and *vitalism* may be in terms of *vitalism's self-organization.* When we contemplate in our own species, the beginnings of life for each of us from the moment of conception, the fertilized cell, that first cell dividing into two; it in turn dividing into four and so on, until a small ball of cells, the *mulberry,* is formed. Then these begin their journey of differentiation.

Which brings us to ask ourselves the question: what is the motivating power, the guiding force, the co-ordinating factor, the organizing "brain" that enables this little miracle to take place? How is it possible to dispute the presence within the living organism of a *Vital Force,* a *purposeful, self-regulating* force governing, modifying and utilizing the purely chemical forces of the inorganic world?

I've used some, what I believe to be, key words here; words which are suggestive of an "intelligence". Words which have a profound resonance at the deepest level of my being: words which imply an *organizing principle.* Words which beg the next question: from whence, and from what, does this mystery stem?

Many of you will no doubt have your own ideas and your own interpretations of them. For my part I am content to accept that *Vitalism is*. Period. That it is in our midst undeniably: that it is a *presence*; that without its existence or presence there would be *chaos* as though a bunch of foreign materials had been flung together haphazardly; this is the antithesis of *organization*. And does not the word *organization* suggest *intelligence?*

Whereas isn't it glaringly obvious that the life processes within that microcosm that is each of us, are not, and *cannot be disorganized?*

For a more penetrating insight into a logical extension of these principles – and their application - into our everyday life, we might well refer to some of the teachings to which I was exposed in my very early study days. This was part of the (North American, I may say) Physio-Medical school which comprised entirely of medical doctors and had its zenith in the late 19th and early 20th century.

Among their great advocates was one, J.M. Thurston, MD, who was Professor of Nervous Diseases at the Physio-Medical College, Indiana. In his book, *The Philosophy of Physio-Medicalism*, (1900), he set out what he called his Theorem and Principia, and I want to quote just one extract from this. It reads:

Vital force, through living matter, is always resistive, and reconstructive, in intent and purpose, when the Vital domain is invaded by inimical substances, forces or influences.

What a powerful statement that was - and is. And such beautiful language. Here was Thurston, a towering intellect, saying in effect, that, *even in the presence of the most serious illness, the body's self-correcting and self-regulating mechanisms were still trying to assert their reconstructive capabilities.*

Now isn't that something? No ifs. No buts. In other words, even if all seemed lost, *there continues to be a positive force trying with all its strength to re-assert normality.* We are day and daily assailed by the negatives. "The next Asian 'flu is on the way.....". "The prognosis is not encouraging....." "He will have to retire from the game with that recurring injury...."

Might it not be just possible that, if the body's healing flow – *previously locked up* – were to be released, the problem may just be resolved?

From within outwards.

There is little evidence in the world of medicine of any awareness that the healing *thrust* of the forces within the body's own system is positive. That these forces are always towards *protection* of the system. They are *never* towards disorder.

So that, if disorder appears on the horizon, we are being warned that those protective mechanisms are compromised in some way and to varying degrees. Disorganization has reared its ugly head and the body's own inherent re-organization forces are needed.

Let's call in the cavalry.

It's called ***movement***.

If we are prepared to look a little deeper into that mysterious world of physiology it becomes clear that life in the organic world – including our own species – had one phenomenon in common.

That commonality is ***movement*** and not only movement in the voluntary sense of the word, but *movement* at the involuntary level. Physiology implies *movement* – respiration, cardiac function, blood flow, cerebrospinal fluid fluctuation, fluids crossing the membranous walls of cells *are all aspects of* ***movement***.

Nothing living in nature is static.

Life processes demand ***movement***.

The most significant characteristic of living processes is ***movement***.

Movement is a primary, even primal, component of the life-providing principles of both the animal and vegetable kingdoms.

But we must remember that it is ***movement*** which finally allows the organism to reach its *maximum level of function*. If we add to this the concept of the Vital or Life Force, where the word *force* is defined as, ***strength*** or ***intense effort***, we can begin to see a formulation emerging.

It is the ability, or otherwise, of the organism to produce the *intense* effort, ***from within***, which will, in turn, determine how well we are functioning. The requirement is to free the organism's ability to raise its function to its maximum potential. As we shall see, ***movement*** becomes the key factor in determining the level at which we are ticking over.

We must also remind ourselves that *all true healing is centrifugal.* And while there are occasions when it is necessary for health issues to be addressed *centripetally* – emergency surgery, for example – in the main, it is from *inside outwards* that the *healing flow* will take place and it is that flow that the true healer must facilitate,

Movement, then, becomes a major facilitator of ***organization***, and *organization* itself is a *distinctive characteristic of the vitalistic principle.*

There cannot be a vitalistic expression without organization.

It was this increasing realisation of the significance of ***movement*** in conjunction with the Vitalistic principle, that spurred me to further exploration. If ***movement*** was a factor in the health delivery process, the next question seemed to be: *how much* ***movement***? It seemed logical that the *quantity* of ***movement*** would play a part. There had to be an optimum *level* of ***movement*** for full function. Anything less is strictly dys-function, even if there are no recognisable, or apparently obvious, signs of dysfunction - symptoms.

For example, if the full quantity of blood flowing to a particular area should be potentially, say level 10 on the scale of functionality, then by simple conclusion, if it is less than that, it is *abnormal.* If the blood supply *to* your liver is less than level 10, then the actual tissue substance of that organ will be deprived of blood and, therefore, nutrition. It will follow then that the ability of the organ to fulfil its mission will be compromised.

It's not exactly rocket science, is it?

These same principles apply throughout the body. And let us not forget that all these myriad functions being carried out every second of the day over our lifetimes are not self-contained within that tissue, or organ, or that system. They are not labouring away in their own little corners to the exclusion of everything else going on in the other corners. Everything is inter-connected. Everything is inter-dependent.

Everything is organized.

But nothing stays still in that continuing process of organization.

We are most decidedly, therefore, a collection of parts, perhaps vaguely connected in some way – a kidney, a shoulder, a toe, an eye, a lung and so on. We are the most incredible composite of organized, integrated functionality and every player in this microcosm which constitutes each of us cannot play alone.

The violin alone cannot produce Beethoven's Fifth. Nor can the flautist. Nor can the French Horn. It has to be a symphony of all of the components. And even that would be chaos without the ***Conductor***.

Who, or what, then, is the ***Conductor*** in this little miracle of the life

Chapter 3.

The Involuntary Mechanism

We have what we seek. It is there all the time, and if we give it time it will make itself known to us.
Thomas Merton

Over the years, medicine has become more and more fragmented. Some would say diversified. Some would say specialised. And who would argue that there have not been benefits to us all from these processes? Unfortunately, one result is that we have begun increasingly to look for answers to the mainstream of health problems myopically.

We are looking at what are believed to be the sub microscopic *irregularities*, or *effects*, of disorders in the increasing expectation that all will be revealed and explained. The secrets behind a wide range of disorders are being portrayed as having their origins in layers of our make-up far removed not only from our vision but even more so, from beyond our comprehension.

We are daily assailed with the latest new "exciting", "promising" or "potentially significant" research for a wide range of illnesses and disorders. The public relations machine can be very persuasive. Each illness or disease – I'll call them all *disorders* to simplify things – is regarded as a little self-contained "compartment" to which we give a name.

The totality of the patient has been relegated in favour of the parts.

Thus, we have our psoriasis patients; then there might be our gall bladder ones; then there are our duodenal ulcer ones; then our sciatica ones. And so on. The list of possibilities is virtually endless.

Those names of disorders and illnesses are descriptions, and classifications, of symptoms and symptom patterns. They may refer to a location in the body, such as the knee, the finger, the chest. Or, they may refer to something more generalised, as in "these swellings on my fingers and stiffness in my neck". Or, maybe just something functional as in, "my back aches and I can hardly move".

For the most part, these symptom patterns are regarded as disorders *in themselves* and largely divorced from any other part of the body. They are perceived, and thought of, as the *target*, effectively a self-contained compartment and largely divorced from all the other compartments. They are ring fenced.

Why? Because, can't you see, that's what the patient is complaining about? Ergo, that's what we treat, that thing there!

In this scenario the belief is that disorder A (having been identified with a name) = procedure A, be it drugs, surgery, chemo or whatever else. It is the area where symptoms have arisen. The symptoms have to be addressed, not the patient.

There is an urgent need to move away from symptomatic treatment - the practice both of waiting for symptoms to arise and, when they do, of addressing them as if they were *the* disorder. This has led us up the blind alley of believing that there is, and will continue to be, a never-ending stream of improved approaches for the ever expanding names of disorders. Having said that, I am happy to acknowledge that there have been considerable improvements in such areas as surgery, much of it technologically driven.

But I'm here referring to that generality of disorders which ought to be amenable to conservative treatment. Alas, I see not the slightest sign that this will happen and for a number of reasons. One of them is the corruptive influence of money. But the other, and probably most important of all, is that there is little likelihood of medicine re-visiting its philosophical roots and going back to the drawing board.

It's as if, somewhere back near the beginning, medicine came to the Y-fork, took the chemical road and, as the years have elapsed since, finds itself diverging further and further away from the most wonderful self-regulating chemical laboratory of all – the human body. From this there developed the apparently spectacular *chemical manipulation* of that wonderful laboratory. It proceeds apace to this day and masquerades under the name of "healthcare".

So where did the other fork in the road go? Much of it went in varying degrees along the vitalistic road, to which I've already referred. Some of it has been invaluable, some not. But I invite you to join me on a journey of both exploration and logic which, I believe, has already transformed healthcare delivery substantially. Let's see what we can see when we stand back and look at the Big Picture.

* * * *

The history of medicine is full of landmarks ranked as milestones in the pursuit of further knowledge in the field. Some names such as Pasteur, the plagiarist of Bechamp, would rank zero with me but, among those whose names would be acknowledged, for example, is that of Andreas Vesalius, the Belgian anatomist. Surprisingly, no one knew much about anatomy until 1543 when Vesalius wrote *De Humani Corporis Fabrica, Libri Septem (On the Structure of the Human Body, in Seven Books).*

Also ranking high in the pecking order would be the English physician William Harvey's discovery in 1628 of what the heart does and how the blood circulates. Nowhere, however, that I am aware of, is the name William Garner Sutherland to be found among the Greats, and I predict that his name will eventually be listed as one of the greatest.

William Garner Sutherland, DO, (1873-1954), is credited as being the originator of osteopathy in the cranial field, commonly known as Cranial Osteopathy. He became a student of Dr Andrew Taylor Still, the founder of Osteopathy. Sutherland was intrigued with the concepts of structure and function and one day, the story goes, he looked at the bones of a skull (there are 22 of these in all) lying on Still's desk. He pondered the make up of these, particularly where they are joined one to the other (called sutures), and noticed that these, in order to articulate one with the other, appeared "like gills of a fish".

He finally concluded that these sutures – like hinges, or seams - were designed for ***motion***. We are reminded that, in all anatomical books, these sutures in adulthood are described as "fused". No movement. That remains the consensus to this day, including, I may say, within the mainstream of the Osteopathic community and beyond.

When Sutherland put his thoughts of the potential for ***motion*** to his teacher, Still replied, "It has to, to be able to accommodate for ***movement***."

Sutherland was positing to himself the theory that if the bones of the skull were designed for ***motion***, then restrictions to ***motion*** would inhibit health. For a number of years, he worked quietly exploring and developing his theories and by 1946, Sutherland's work had attracted a considerable interest and following.

Cranial motion can be defined as a rhythmic motion in which all 22 bones of the head move cyclically between two poles and during which fluid pressure increases and decreases alternately within one cycle. The brain, blood vessels and cerebrospinal fluid take part in these pressure changes.

By any standards Sutherland's assertion was extraordinary. It was also courageous and challenging, as the received wisdom of the day and which remains the standard teaching to this day is – no movement. In the cadaver, the cranial bones are fused.

Nevertheless, his work was taken up by others, such as Harold I. Magoun, Sr., DO, (1898-1981), who was one of Sutherland's early students and author of *Osteopathy in the Cranial Field*. Others included such names as Robert Fulford, DO, author of *Touch of Life and Philosopher, Physician*, Beryl E. Arbuckle, DO, whose *Selected Writings* bring into sharp focus the impact of the birthing processes on the infant and, not least, Denis Brookes, DO, PhD, author of *Lectures in Cranial Osteopathy,* and who was my own teacher.

There were many others, all contributing to the knowledge base that was developing, about the role of the cranial dimension in the health and disease processes. The techniques associated with cranial osteopathy, and its derivatives, also evolved in a similar fashion to that from which it spawned – Osteopathy. The early adherents and researchers in this new field were highly motivated and many of them saw this new player on the stage as promising major strides in the health delivery processes. However, while reports of results began to mount, they were largely modest and, to an extent, anecdotal over a period of (currently) some 60 years.

There was also what some considered to be another problem. If there was ***movement*** - motion - of the cranial bones, how can this be demonstrated? Where is the research? Where is the proof? At this time, I am aware of research which claims to "prove" there is cranial motion, and research which claims the opposite. Perhaps one of the most interesting commentaries comes in an article published courtesy of *NASA's Space Operations Mission Directorate* in 2004:

NASA has developed a type of ultrasound method to monitor intracranial pressure by measuring the subtle movements of the skull. Most people think the skull is a rigid container that doesn't change in size or volume. It's been shown, however, that the skull moves with changes in Intra Cranial Pressure (pressure within the head). The movement is so small that it is not even detectable to the human eye. The movement is only a few micrometers—and it takes 1,000 micrometers to make 1 millimetre.

The call for proof of an *involuntary* movement is, I believe, now redundant. The question really needs to be something like this:

How is it possible for there to be life processes ***in the absence of an involuntary moving mechanism****?*

Medicine, conventional or otherwise, has evolved over centuries in the absence of any awareness both of the existence, and ***even more importantly, of the significance of***

an involuntary controlling mechanism. The implication is that we are essentially *static* organisms which nevertheless manifest ***movement or moving phenomena*** from a fixed baseline.

There has not, and never has been, to my knowledge, a suggestion that behind and underpinning any of the bodily activities which include *movement* – and what activity does not? – there exists a mechanism which is itself both a moving one *and the source of all other movements, both at the voluntary and involuntary level.*

At least not until the arrival of Dr Sutherland.

It seems quite inconceivable that those moving activities which constitute the presence of the body's life forces can themselves function in the presence of an otherwise *static* organism and, from which it must logically follow, that there must be an organizing or controlling self-perpetuating or self-propelling source. It would be at once self-contained and the driver of all functions.

It is readily apparent that, until there is recognition and acknowledgement of the existence and role of such a mechanism, there will continue to have major limitations imposed on medicine's declared quest to *conquer* the vast array of challenges that continue in this area. As currently constituted present day research is mainly pharmaceutically or technology driven, the limitations of which are for all to see. A change of direction from these entrenched sources, however, is unlikely for obvious reasons.

There is no doubt in my own mind but that *there is* ***cranial motion***, that it is probably in a form originally described by Sutherland as rhythmic and alternating, and that it has a very significant impact on the body's life processes. The only question remaining relates to the significance, or otherwise, of that ***movement*** in relation to our health and wellbeing.

Further, fusion of the sutures of the cranial bones would not only prevent ***motion*** in a *physiological* sense and, therefore, prevent any alternating and intra cranial pressure changes taking place. It would also disallow any possibility of changes taking place in the *anatomical* relationship of any cranial bone with its contiguous bones. Fusion is fusion. Rigid is rigid. In short, the "shape" of an adult head, in total, would then be unalterable, if sutures were fused.

Such is manifestly not the case and is easily demonstrable and is visible to the naked eye, given the application of the specific and relevant techniques.

Chapter 4.

Birthing

Our birth is nothing but our death begun.
Edward Young

Most, if not all, practitioners in the cranial field agree that our entry into this world, and indeed the developing processes within the womb before then, have a significant influence on the cranial structures. You may be surprised to learn that that even applies to those of us who have arrived through caesarean section. And so we must go back to when our journeys all began.

Sutherland referred to the moving cranial mechanism as the body's Primary Respiratory Mechanism (PRM). It was a primary *physiological* process, just as is blood circulation, lymph drainage, kidney filtration or any of the body's other living processes. The word "primary" was to signal his belief that the movement was just that – primary, or essential, to the body's life processes. The word "respiratory" was to describe an ebb and flow phenomenon akin to normal breathing.

This ebb and flow, in practice, was constituted by alternating pressure changes within the head, in which there was a phase of increased pressure followed by a phase of decrease. Some think of it as a pumping action. It can be likened to a sine wave as in Figure 1.

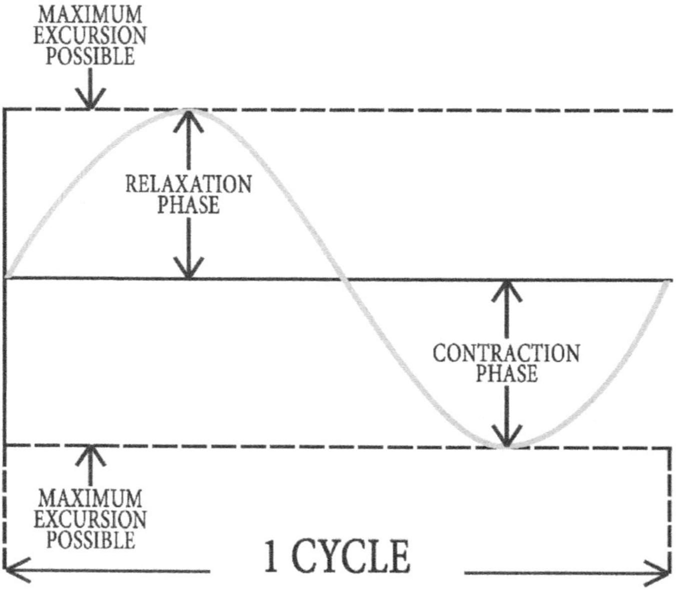

Fig. 1

Thus, we have ***motion*** extending over our lifetimes from the time of our arrival (and before) until the time of our departure. It became clear that the physical *act* of our arrival was no ill-thought-out exercise either.

The *act* itself had *purpose.*

In a normal birthing delivery, the head travels through the birth canal, during which journey the very malleable little bones of the head are compressed. On exiting the canal these soft bones, and the as yet open sutures, *blow out* due to the normal forces and pressures within the head wanting to make as much room within it as possible. The *decompression* event.

So, is this all-sheer accident? Or is it by design? This is a philosophical, rather than a scientific or medical, question. The answer is abundantly clear. Think of it like this. In the old days before you, dear reader, were born, it used to be common practice on a cold morning to have to jump start the car. Out came the starting handle, insert it into the whatsitsname, give it a few swings and, bingo, there was life.

I think of this scenario when I think of the birthing process. The very *act* of the *compression, squashing* of the cranial bones within the birth canal, is itself the preparation for the explosive act of *decompression* of these bones – the blowing out. Together these forces are the kick start to the life processes of the infant.

And here's another thing. Why blow out? The answer is that nature has decreed that the space within that little head should be maximized from the outset. (You may have noticed that many politicians have not had this experience!). The birthing act itself, therefore, has not only the *purpose* of transferring the infant to the outside world, but of preparing it, *as part of the same process,* for maximum *function*. And who would complain about getting two for one? The economy and purpose of nature combined with intent. Genius.

Where, then, does that leave our little babes who arrive abnormally? They would be mainly those arriving by caesarean section, a procedure which is increasingly commonplace in Western society. The reasons for this are various, ranging from mothers who are "too posh to push", through a belief that it's best for Junior, to malpractice fearing physicians and to those occasions when it is medically necessary.

Whatever the reasons, there is a general belief that caesarean section deliveries are less traumatic on the infant (and mother) and, therefore, should be considered as a preferred birthing method. However, except in those cases where it is deemed medically necessary, it is otherwise a downside.

Over the years I've been practising, I began to notice that, in the case of children who came to me as patients, my questioning of the parent in relation to the circumstances of the birth was producing a pattern. The major categories of disorder of my paediatric patients have been mainly in areas such as asthma, infantile eczema, cerebral palsy, autism and attention deficit, among others.

In the absence of supporting data, it began to emerge that the majority of these children had been caesarean births. The percentage of caesarean births in the population as a whole is somewhere in the 25% range of all births, yet the incidence of disorders in my paediatric patients was far in excess of this figure. It should have been something like 1 in 4, caesarean to normal. Instead, I estimate it was more like 3 to 1.

Ongoing conventional medical research has also noticed. In a report in the online journal, *Diabetologia* (2008), it was reported that studies of Type 1 diabetes in children revealed that those delivered by caesarean section were at 20% greater risk of suffering from the condition.

The researchers said that "*...the reason for this is still not understood, though it is possible that the caesarean section itself is responsible, perhaps because babies born via that method are first exposed to bacteria from the hospital environment rather than to maternal bacteria*".

I confess I would have reservations about the suggested possible reasons given and would be of the opinion that a more likely possibility is the deprivation of those infant heads to the *compression* and *decompression* phenomenon.

In a study published in *The Journal of Pediatrics* in 2008, the authors concluded that, "*Compared to children born in the natural way (i.e. spontaneously and vaginally), children born by Caesarean section had an approximately 50 % increased risk of developing asthma*". They also concluded that, "*Children born vaginally, but with assistance from vacuum or forceps, had a 20 % increased risk of asthma*".

Let's now look at some of the practical implications of these matters on our health over the ensuing years.

Chapter 5.

Cranial Injury

There is nothing more frightful than ignorance in action.
Goethe

There are two other major problems in determining what will happen to the infant head as part of its entry into this world.

The first concerns the relative balance of tensions of the structures within the pelvic area of mother. The womb is essentially a muscular organ, served and supported by an array of ligaments. All muscles contract and relax in varying degrees so that, in theory, those of the womb should be in a sustained state of relaxation throughout the pregnancy and therefore conveying that easy balance of muscular tensions on Junior during the period of development.

Such is rarely the case. As we shall see, that full state of muscular relaxation – of all organs and systems - is absent in just about every one of us at any given point in time in our lives, and in varying degrees throughout the body. It just so happens that we are here particularly concerned with a major female reproductive organ which has the no mean task of nurturing us during the growth through pregnancy, before bringing us into the world.

That's the state of affairs *within* the womb. The second concern revolves around the *delivery* processes themselves – what happens after we leave the womb. Right away, let me say that we are into an area where many questions remain unanswered but here are a few of the reasons suggested for some of the difficulties that arise. I must add that I claim no obstetric skills or training:

1. Forceps delivery and vacuum extractions. Let us recall that Junior has already made the first stage of the journey into the birth canal. The head has already been significantly stressed before it arrives at the exit. It will already have been subjected to the muscular tension status *within* the womb, as indicated above. There will also be unequal pressures in the surrounding pelvic floor structures beyond the womb and extending to the birth canal structures themselves. These unequal pressures – imbalances - surrounding the birth canal are then further imposed on that little head during its journey. Remember, at this time those very fragile and malleable bones are capable of being twisted any old which-way. It's a miracle Junior is still with us by this time. Which demonstrates, of course, the degree to which the life forces can operate, even when the system is under duress.

And then comes the final physical insult. We apply the forceps or vacuum extraction to something *which is already under stress* and, without having a notion that there is a critical part played by those cranial structures in the body's life producing mechanisms. Indeed, there is no awareness that there is even such a thing as *a mechanism.*

2. The second problem is probably more to do with our western culture.

Our entry into this world was designed so that the associated forces applied to the head ***would be from the top downwards****, not the reverse.*

Even without the use of aids, such as forceps, and with nothing more than manual assistance, the infant's head again commonly becomes subject to the arbitrary stresses and strains imposed by the hands of a medical operator. All of these stresses will exert a *pull* on the head and will be invasive in varying degrees. The one, however, which is most likely of all to be injurious is where the operator exerts a pulling force to the bone at the back of the head.

All of the above procedures result in the direction of forces being applied to the head in the ***opposite*** *direction to those required and designed by nature.*

This can have the most negative effect on the *anatomical* relationship of the cranial bones, one with the other. As an aside, I recall sometime in 1978, I believe, seeing the movie *Centennial*, based on the book of the same name by James Michener. The movie was set in the pioneering days of the American West in a fictional town in Colorado. This was also about the same time that I first became interested in cranial work. One particular scene struck me forcibly.

In this, a North American native squaw was giving birth to her baby and, contrary to the bed position adopted by western women, the squaw was in the squat position with her arms draped over a horse tethering rail. How natural it all seemed for both mother and child. Why, I wondered, do we not adopt such obviously simple and natural practices in our society?

The effect now of these contrary forces on the head, and at the beginning of the life of the infant, is to produce *distorted relationships in the position of the bones with each other*. In other words, the bones of the head are not in symmetry. Examples of this can be seen all around you and, often enough, in the mirror! Have a look at your TV presenters, personalities, your friends (I recommend you don't let them know what you're up to, lest you want to lose them, of course). Here's some of what you will see even with the untrained eye:

On the horizontal plane of the head – and allowing for any tilt of the head sideways – does one eye look lower than the other? In fact, does your own head tend to be tilted sidewise, usually to the one side?

Or, does one eye seem smaller than the other?

Is one ear lower than the other?

Does one ear look farther forward in the head than the other?

Do the teeth look off centre in the mouth?

These abnormalities – and many more - are all commonly observed around us in everyday life once you are aware of what to look for. They are easily observed indications of the *imperfections* of the bony alignment which had their origins back at birth, and before. These are *imperfections* of the anatomy of the head and the question then arises: so what?

Let's not forget that these *asymmetrically* aligned bones are all the while to-ing and fro-ing as part of the body's absolutely *essential* life processes – ***movement***. It is like a pumping action, an ongoing expansion and contraction. As we have seen in Figure 1, that ***movement*** is designed to allow the <u>*maximum*</u> peaks and troughs of pressure change within the head. The ***movement*** itself takes place about the joints –

sutures – between each of these 22 bones. What then happens to those alternating pressure changes *in the presence of bones which are misaligned, warped, twisted, torqued?*

It's pretty obvious, isn't it? They are doing their best to open up, then close, open up and close to the best of their ability, *even in the presence of a warp, a twist - an impediment – in their way, caused by the restrictions to free movement in the sutures,* due to the torque of all 22 bones. And ALL of the bones are always involved, even if some are in greater degrees of limited movement than others. It's never just one or two or more bones, while the rest are okay. It can't be. It's the composite whole.

Instead, therefore, of the Primary Respiratory Mechanism going full blast, as in Figure 1, we have a range of variants, all of which are *resulting from* the flaws in the alignment of the bones of the head (cranial bones). Examples of these are shown in Figures, 2, 3 and 4. Please note, however, that these examples are theoretical and are given for illustrative purposes only.

The main points to note are that there are significant departures from normal (maximum contraction and relaxation) in all cases, but also that each is different from the others. None of our "abnormalities" is exactly the same as anyone else's.

There is already dysfunction to the body's life processes.

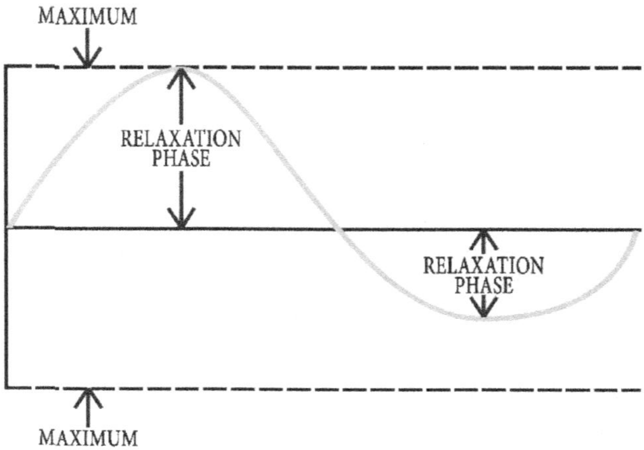

ABNORMALITY IS INABILITY TO REACH FULL AMPLITUDE IN ONE PHASE ONLY

Fig. 2

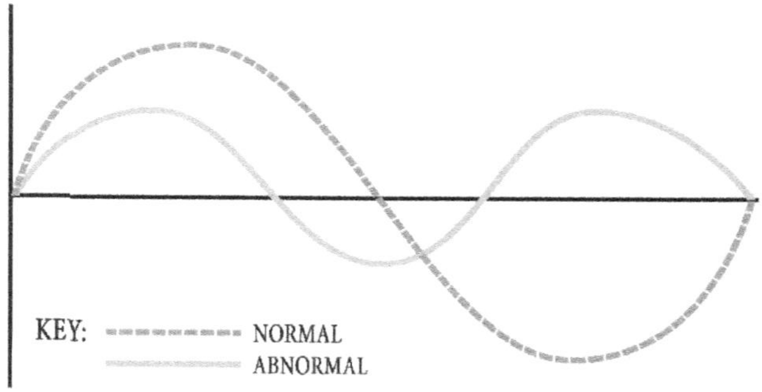

ABNORMALITY IS THAT BOTH CONTRACTION AND RELAXATION PHASES ARE REDUCED IN AMPLITUDE AND CYCLE FREQUENCY

Fig. 3

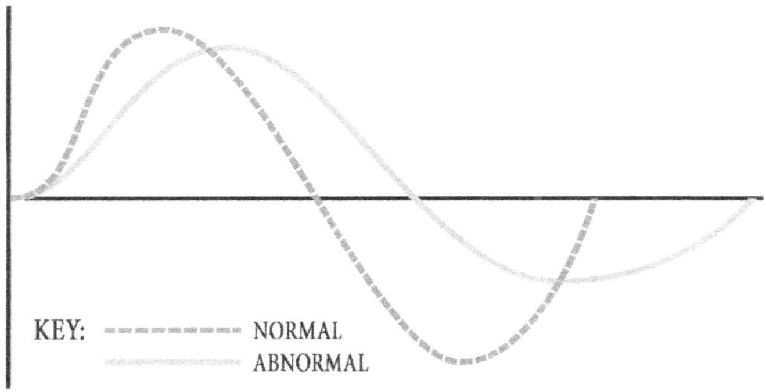

Fig.4

Departures from normal are present with each of us, but this does not mean that each of us is "ill" in the normal understanding of the word. Far from it in many cases. We mostly (hopefully) are walking around free of symptoms. I'm often struck by the body's ability to apparently carry on, in the presence of a variety of inherent challenges.

What it does mean, however, is that the basic level of functioning of the life processes is below par. They are not up to full speed. They are not firing on all cylinders. They constitute an inherent and inbuilt weakness in the system which then ***predisposes*** the system to respond to other, mostly external, factors which, in practice, almost always get the blame for the abnormalaties.

This becomes a permanent and fixed ***weakness*** *present throughout life.*
Let me give you some examples:

1. Lucy is driving the car, a child dashes on to the road, she steps really hard on the brakes and, bingo, a pain shoots through her lower back and she's virtually immobilised. A very simple act. Question: did she twist "awkwardly"? Did she "knock something out"? Was there some kind of weakness there beforehand that she didn't know about? Or did the sudden shock to the system play a part?

2. John starts to notice that, after eating, he is getting the occasional indigestion type pain. He modifies his diet on the advice of his pal, Paul. This helps for a while but, after a time, he finds he needs to resort to using antacid medications which quickly take care of the problem. Then it recurs and gets worse. Eventually, however, he seeks professional help and is diagnosed to have a tumour. Question: was his fondness for the occasional hot and spicy food the cause? After all, he didn't go overboard and he knew a lot of people whose diets were a lot worse than his? Or, maybe it was the ten a day smoking in his youth and early twenties? Or, was there some other weakness there beforehand, bubbling along in the background that he didn't know about?

3. Jane started to feel some stiffness in her joints – hands, fingers, shoulders – to the extent that she had to resort to painkilling medications. Finally, her doctor diagnosed rheumatoid arthritis. Question: Aunt Liz had it, so I suppose it's in the

family? Or, it started soon after that awful 'flu she had last year. I wonder, did that cause it? Or, maybe there is some other weakness that's behind these headaches, heart issues and so on, that have been dogging her more and more?

4. Little Pete has been getting more and more out of control. He's lost all concentration, is restless, is tyrannising his teacher and now they want to put him on to Ritalin. Question: is this an inherited thing? Or, is there something here going back to that pretty horrendous birth?

There is a strong probability that, behind the scenes in each of these cases, we will find an underlying, and significant, weakness in the ability of the system to perform the myriad of tasks which go to make up the *composite* of functions and which constitute *balance*. Normality.

Certainly, all of these stories can, and often do, have other influences which are relevant to the onset of the symptoms. Or, at least, recognisable symptoms. In example 1 above, for example, we note that Lucy stepped hard on the brake and, so we conclude that the *act* of the swift and hard step somehow or other was the cause. Maybe the speed of her reaction was the cause? Maybe she part twisted in the process? In practice, however, these will have been *secondary* causes. They will have been *contributory* causes and, indeed, had Lucy not reacted as she did, it is probable that nothing would have resulted to her.

More than likely, though, there would have been something similar when next week, next month or next year she loaded up the car with the heavy box of wines from the supermarket. Or when she reached that heavy power drill to husband John up the ladder. You get the picture? Lucy's back problem was *triggered* by an act – it could be any act – because there was an *inherent* and largely *silent* weakness there *beforehand*, just waiting to be brought to the surface. After all, when you come to think about it, it hardly makes much sense when a simple act sets in motion such a severe reaction, does it? The body can't be as fragile as that.

And it isn't, *if it is free of any significant predisposing weaknesses.*

It is almost always the coming together of two levels of the causative processes which finally result in the problem as recognised by the patient:

predisposing weakness + the precipitating event = a problem.

In practice, in today's society and, believing as we do, *that the symptom is the problem*, many approaches are targeted at the *problem* which is *usually a result, or effect,* rather than a *primary cause.* Admittedly though, many of these are helpful in varying degrees in targeting the *effect.*

And so, the painkiller may help the pain; the surgery may help the gall stones; the mobilisation of the lumbar spine may help the sciatica; and the root canal procedure may help the abscess on the tooth. Further, however long it might take, the symptoms might remain clear for a long time and maybe forever. But then it might not.

The question remaining, however, is this:

If the effect (symptoms) has gone, has the ***cause*** *been addressed?*

In none of the cases listed above has there been evidence of a cause having been addressed. Symptoms were targeted. There was breakdown and yet, short of something like a fall from the tenth floor, or mistakenly drinking the garden weedkiller, we are wondrously made and in theory should not be so easily succumbing to a vast array of disorders which we see day and daily around us.

But then as we've seen, there is with all of us an underlying factor which few are aware of. It is this phenomenon which is the real culprit. If we can do something about it - ***and the first need is to recognise that it is even there*** - then we dramatically alter the equation in the patient's favour. If we can change the basic functionality level from, say, 5.5 on the scale to, say, 8.2, or whatever else it can be, the body's integration, co-ordination, organization - its wholeness – are changed forever. Why, then, would it ever breakdown to the same degree again in the future *when the underlying level of function is so much better?*

Chapter 6.

The Dura Mater

The great affair is to move...
Robert Louis Stevenson

I've referred a lot to ***movement***, or motion. So, what is there about this phenomenon that ranks it so important to us in the world of healing and healthcare?

Somewhere back in the mists of time it became clear that life in the organic world – including our own species – had one phenomenon in common. That commonality was ***movement***.

So that,

MOVEMENT = LIFE
NO MOVEMENT = DEATH

Simple as that.

I guess that was what first attracted me to explore this Primary Respiratory Mechanism (PRM) of Dr Sutherland, and about which I had begun increasingly to hear. Finally, and after much time and research of my own, it was as clear that Sutherland's PRM was effectively not only a major key to the life processes, but was ***the*** major key to sustaining ***all of the body's life processes***.

This was the crucial mechanism. And yet, to this day, its very existence is scarcely known about. Remarkable, to say the least.

I began to see that ***movement***, in its widest sense, is a primary component of the life-providing principles of both the animal and vegetable kingdoms.

There is never an absence of movement in the presence of organic life.

Sometimes it is massive, as when the plates of our planet shift. Even when they are apparently still, there continues to be ***movement*** in the ground below our feet. Then there is growth. The grass beneath our feet grows, as do the trees above our heads, even if interrupted by the temporary repose of the seasons or even the apparent repose of hibernation. The universe around us is never still. Then there is the wind; and there are the expansions and contractions of day and night, heat and cold. Even when other materials such as water, oxygen and nutrients are also needed for the sustenance of life, ***movement*** is still central to the processes.

If, therefore, ***movement*** is the driving force to just about all those things that make us tick, the question then was: where is the engine to drive this ***movement***? What is the mechanism? In what way does it manifest? How does it affect the body's function?

I've referred previously to the question of *proof* of the existence of this ***movement***. It is many years now since the suggestion was first posited about the presence of an involuntary mechanism of primary importance to health and welfare. And yet, perhaps surprisingly, there continues to be little evidence of any interest in such a mechanism from within the world of conventional medicine. But then, why should there be? Research is expensive and most, therefore, have strings attached. There has to be an investment return and so those who control most of it continue to feed into the chemical road at the Y-fork. After all, that's where all the answers will be found.

It's no surprise, therefore, to find that research in this area is limited and restricted to specific purposes and needs, such as we have found in the NASA paper. The technology is already available to measure the *existence* of ***cranial movement***, and the ability to determine pressure changes within the head. What is now needed is a recognition of the importance of that ***movement***, not only in space exploration, but in the generality of health provision.

Definitions might here be in order:

scientific fact

Definition: *any observation that has been repeatedly confirmed and accepted as true; any scientific observation that has not been refuted*

Webster's New Millennium™ Dictionary of English, Preview Edition.

Sir James Paget (1814-1899), the British physician, after whom Paget's Disease is named, noted "That which is clinically proved needs no other evidence." Within the meaning of the foregoing definition, the understandings behind the philosophy of the ***Bio Craniopathy*** are now well established, as are the results which are "repeatedly confirmed".

There is no doubt in my mind as to the existence of *cranial motion*, for the simple reason that, if it did not exist, there would be no changes to the health status of patients for whom ***Bio Craniopathy*** is used. The results are often both observable, in terms of changes in the person's anatomy (relative eye levels, for example) and measurable by simple tests such as in Applied Kinesiology. They can also be seen from standard laboratory tests such as for blood sugar level changes, blood pressure checks and monitoring of cholesterol levels.

But let's not get ahead (excuse the pun!) of ourselves. What we need to look at now are the bits and pieces which go to make up the *engine*. For that's exactly what the Primary Respiratory Mechanism is – the engine upon which just about virtually every activity depends.

That means not only the pretty obvious things like how well you walk or how easily you kick the ball. But also how well all of the body's constituent parts right down to cellular level, and beyond, are performing. For example, how efficiently are the kidneys filtering the wastes out of the blood. Each day, your kidneys process about 200 quarts of blood to sift out about 2 quarts of waste products and extra water. And you didn't even have to think about.

Then, what about, say, the pancreas? What is it doing? Well, many things, including completing the work of breaking down protein, carbohydrates, and fats using digestive juices of pancreas combined with juices from the intestines.

Even at the cellular level there is activity; there is function; there is ***movement***. No one knows how many of the little players there are, but an approximate number would be in the order of 100 trillion. Their activity is *organized*: it is intelligently *purposeful*.

And with these examples, we are looking at a mere miniscule of all of the functions carried out by these structures and *upon which life depends.* This ***constantly moving mechanism***, the PRM, then, is the ***source** of function*, the source of physiology, the *controller* of everything that goes together to allow you to read (or hear) these words. The engine, in effect.

And, did you ever know of an engine that didn't have its own very special casing? I can't think of one, though I'm no engineer. The casing of an engine has a specific purpose. That being to facilitate the *functioning* of the engine and, usually to *protect* the mechanism.

We're back to rocket science again, aren't we?

What, then, would happen if the casing were to be somehow damaged? Even slightly? Maybe a few dents? Maybe something of a twist? That would certainly make some impact on the smooth running of the engine and not for the better, wouldn't it?

And with that analogy, we have our very own casing. It's called the skull. Or, cranium.

The main purpose of the skull is generally believed to be that of protection. Which it obviously does. It comprises a hard and bony structure which encases the all-important brain and also supports major structures such as the eyes, nose, ears and mouth. But it does more than that, as we shall see presently when we consider our old friend ***movement***.

There is no dispute as to the importance of the cranium's protective function. Inside is the brain, universally recognised as probably the single most important organ in the body. Why else would we have the helmets for cyclists, motor cyclists, rugby players, footballers, construction sites and similar.

Its other function – of partaking in a rhythmic ***movement*** – is barely recognised at all. And yet, in my view,

it is the most important function of all taking place in the body.

And, if that is true, what happens to our bodily engine *if the casing is bent, warped or torqued?*

Let's firstly have a look at this protective casing. We are going to have a look at a real skull who (or is it which?) goes by the name of "Henry". In figures 5 and 6, one of the first things to catch the eye are the zig-zag lines in both. These are the joints – the *sutures* – between the bones and, about which the ***respiratory movement*** takes place.

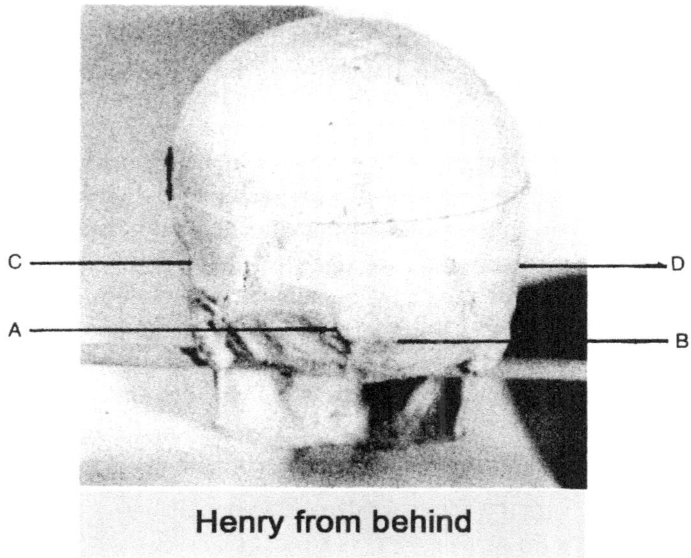

Figure 5. Henry from behind

In figure 5 we are looking at the back of the head, horizontally, and, in the foreground and just about in the middle at the bottom, you will see what looks like a small knob. Branching out from the knob you will then see a line curving upwards and sideways, one to the right (B) and one to the left (A).

The one to the right is *lower* than that to the left and, if you look carefully, the bony material below those two lines is also unequal. The right side is lower than the left. You will also see that the right side of the cranium at (D) is farther back than ite equivalent point on the left side (C). All of which means that the cranium is *rotated* clockwise on the plane, back to front, as we look at it. In plain language, it is twisted and the origin of that will go back to birth, or pre-birth.

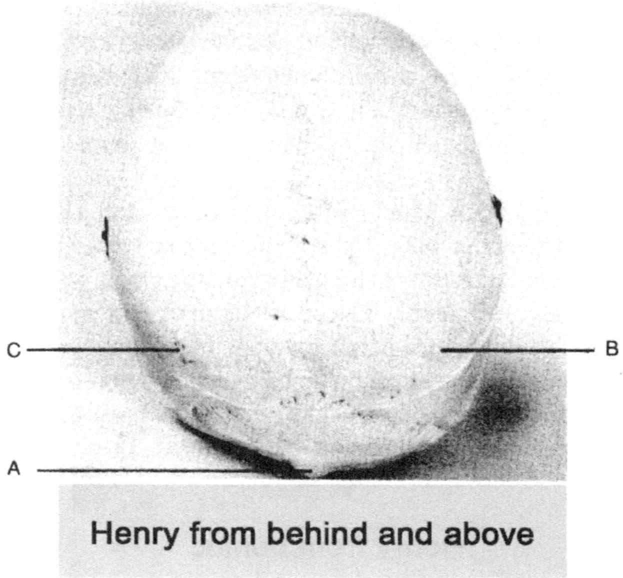

Figure 6. Henry from behind and above.

In Figure 6 you will see the same knob again at the bottom of the picture (A). You will also see on this view that the bony part to the right of the knob (B) effectively a bulge - is further back than that to the left (A). If we were looking down on Henry from directly above, we would see that the skull is *rotated* clockwise on that plane also. Overall, Henry is in a bit of a twist, as are all of us in varying degrees. And that's not the way it was meant to be. All of this will almost certainly have occurred at, or before, birth. Or both.

You will have realised by this time that we have been looking at what the textbooks call *anatomy*. Specifically, that part of our anatomy we refer to as the cranium. I'm here going to refer to another two areas of our anatomy which are vitally important in this scenario of "torqued anatomy" and which are intimately tied in to what we have just seen with Henry.

Never fear, I'm not about to embark on a dissertation on human anatomy. I want to just briefly tie in two other important structures to help complete the circle, as it were. Both are very much linked in to the cranium.

The first of these is the spine which, you will recall, runs from the base of the skull down to the tail bone. It consists of 26 bones, called the vertebrae and the one at the very top, called the *atlas,* physically attaches to the skull. It also moves about its joint with the skull, such as when you move your head or turn your neck.

The second structure is called the ***dura mater***. It's a very strong membrane, part of which is inside the skull and covers the brain. It also *attaches to the inside of the cranial bones themselves.* The rest of the ***dura*** runs down the spinal cord, covering – and protecting – the spinal cord. It finishes up attached to the tailbone. And who hasn't heard of epidurals, especially the ladies?

But this is where things get interesting. Because of the close relationships between these structures - cranium, spine and ***dura mater*** – there is, as you might well imagine, a strong possibility that, whatever happens to one member of this trio, there will result in some spin off into the others. And, indeed, it is so.

Consider this...... Let's get back again to Henry. Here we have a skull which is *rotated variously, twisted, torqued,* All 22 bones are fixed in their various positions one with the other and are all players in this drama. On the inside surfaces of these misaligned bones the poor old ***dura mater*** is attached to them, has nowhere else to go, save to hang in there and play *follow my leader*. And the leader is? The cranium, of course, complete with its torques and twists.

Instead, therefore, of the dural membrane sitting there quietly and at ease with itself, it has had to go with the twist of the cranial bones. It is no longer *at ease*. It is effectively *in tension*, or *contraction,* for the simple reason that is has been forced to bend to the will of Big Brother cranium.

That same level of *contraction* – indeed the whole of the unique tension pattern established by the flawed cranial bones, will then find its way along the continuous strip of the dural membrane, right to the bottom end where it meets the tail bone.

The *tension status* of the ***dura*** is therefore an exact replica, a mirror image in effect, of the state of affairs at the top end which, in turn, is determined by the status of the cranial bones. If you wish to think of the ***dura***, in turn, as being in a twist, that's fine, for essentially that's what it is.

Now, what about the spine? What happens to the vertebrae in this scenario? As well as the first vertebra at the top articulating with the cranium, the ***dural membrane*** throughout the length of the spine actually attaches on to some of the vertebrae. The result, of course, is that the *tension pattern* of the ***dura*** – and let's not forget where, and why, that originated – is *imposed* on the whole of the vertebral column, top to bottom.

Now isn't that something?

Not only that but, if we look at the imbalance at the base of Henry's skull where one side is lower than the other and is also further forward than the other, this means that Henry's first vertebra would have to adjust its position – rotate and sidebend, to use the technical jargon – in order to retain its relationship with the cranium.

Wow, let's take a breather here. Coffee or herbal tea? Coming right up.

As I was saying, we started with birthing; then we saw the resultant impact it had on the alignment of the bones of the head and with just about all of us. And from there, on the bones of the spine.

The ***dura mater*** (Latin for tough mother) might be the *tough mother* but she has to do as she's told by the *higher authority* – the cranium. She has to *adapt* to what is the state of affairs at the cranium. No argument here. There are no compromises in this scenario. The cranium is the ultimate authority – the Chairman and CEO.

And this Chairman knows no bounds, for the next casualty is the spine. Those tensions *imposed* on the spine, *both from the **dural** tensions and directly from the vertebral contact with the cranium* produce the effect of **all vertebrae having to *adapt* to the tensions, stresses, originating from the cranium**.

In other words we have misalignment of the spine *primarily resulting from the need for the vertebrae to **adapt** to the cranial status.*

*The alignment of the spinal vertebrae is almost always determined by the **alignment of the cranial bones.***

This is the domino effect on the spinal vertebrae, resulting from the status of the cranium.

And this is again where I am happy to give full credit to Dr Sutherland, the father of cranial. He was aware from his own researches that there was a unique relationship between the trio of cranium, dura and the spine. It was something of a system in its own right and he appended the name

Reciprocal Tension Membrane to it to describe the reciprocity between the constituent parts with an emphasis on the membranous component, the ***dura***.

There, I've said it. No going back. These spinal misalignments are frequently mistaken for primary misalignments, rather than *secondary,* or *compensatory,* misalignments. And there is obviously a big difference, particularly when it comes to addressing the associated health issues.

Chapter 7.

Optimal Function

Do not expect to arrive at certainty in every subject which you pursue. There are a hundred things wherein we mortals. . . must be content with probability, where our best light and reasoning will reach no farther.
Isaac Watts

Now that we've had a look at the engine casing, let's have a look at the engine itself. This means we are into the "works", the core mechanism upon which so much depends. The first thing we need to get straight is that, with the obvious exceptions of genetic abnormalities such as spina bifida, Down's syndrome, we are all *potentially perfectly designed.* What we are considering here is why that perfect design *is not perfectly functioning.*

There is no detail missing. All the parts are there.

The kidneys, the liver, the gall bladder, the small intestine and large one are there.

The heart, the lungs, the thyroids, the nerves and all those trillions of little cells are there.

And they are all in the right places too.

And they're all connected up so that nothing is left out.

Isn't it extraordinary, all those bits and pieces, large and small, at the ready and just waiting for instructions? And co-ordinated instructions between them all at that? Not one single player will be left out in this scenario of *inter-dependent, purposeful, organized function.*

Every single atom of every single little cell has *purpose.* In spite of the apparent gains of knowledge in medical science, the truth is that we haven't even begun to touch the depths of the intrinsic nature of the "construction", or function, of Man – and Woman, of course.

Furthermore, the knowledge and discoveries of the researchers are in themselves *fragmented,* focused on the parts and divorced from the *totality* of each individual. It calls to mind the old maxim that "we are in danger of knowing more and more about less and less".

So how do we get back to addressing the *composite* individual? The vast majority of named disorders/ diseases are areas of breakdown, believed to be localised. And, of course, some of these must be addressed accordingly. If we are involved in a car wreck then we may need fractures attended to. Or surgery. Or life support. In the overall statistics of breakdown, however, episodes such as these are a very small proportion of the total of what we might call disorder.

As has already been discussed, most disorders are treated:

1. locally, that is, where the disturbance has arisen. That local area is "targeted" in the belief that the removal of the symptoms – by surgery, medication or

whatever other procedures are deemed appropriate – is the best, and often only, road to recovery.

2. when symptoms arise. This is commonly referred to as symptomatic treatment and is regarded as the body's way of signaling that all is not well. In fact, it usually is the body's way of signaling that the body is *getting beyond not functioning well*, but has arrived at the stage of crying out for help. The red flag is up.

So, back to ***movement*** again. Can you visualize a phenomenon in which every single structure in the body is in a constant and continuing state of ***alternating movement***? The ***movement*** takes place between two poles which we can refer to as ***contraction*** and ***relaxation***.

Let's think, for example, of a sponge and we immerse it into a basin of water. We then squeeze it – contraction – and fluid moves out of it. Next we release it – relaxation – and the fluid moves back into it. We keep repeating these actions and we produce what is effectively a pumping type of action.

Now, substitute the brain, and the other structures inside the cranium, for the sponge. These are all being subjected to this constant pumping action throughout our lifetimes; an ongoing squeezing and release, squeezing and release, which is, of course, the Primary Respiratory Mechanism at work.

"Working for YOU!" No, it's not a re-vamp of the latest political slogan. This is for real. This is what is providing for you all of everything it takes to make you the functioning person you are. As far as it goes, that is.

The output from this engine, determining how well all the bits and pieces are performing, is going to be unquestioningly influenced by the ability, or otherwise, of the PRM to *pump* to its maximum ability; to reach its maximum levels of relaxation and contraction. To fire fully on all cylinders.

You will remember the sine wave in Chapter 1, in which the peaks and troughs of the wave represented the *maximum* excursion it was possible to go in each direction. The trough may be represented by the *squeeze* of the sponge – contraction. The peak will therefore be the release – the relaxation phase.

Now, let's insert into the equation a torqued cranium; any cranium. They are all around us, including our own, of course. For our reference, let's just take a look at a graphic of a skull in Figure 7 below. It will give you some outline of the bones of the cranium and, particularly, of the joints (sutures) between them. This is one area where the all-important ***movement*** takes place.

Suppose we now twist, or torque, such a skull and, as we have already seen in Henry, a real skull, we might have something like the sketch in Figures 8. This malformation is very commonly encountered. In practice, the potential permutations of possible outcomes of torquing are virtually limitless. But, for our present purposes this theoretical example will help to demonstrate the point.

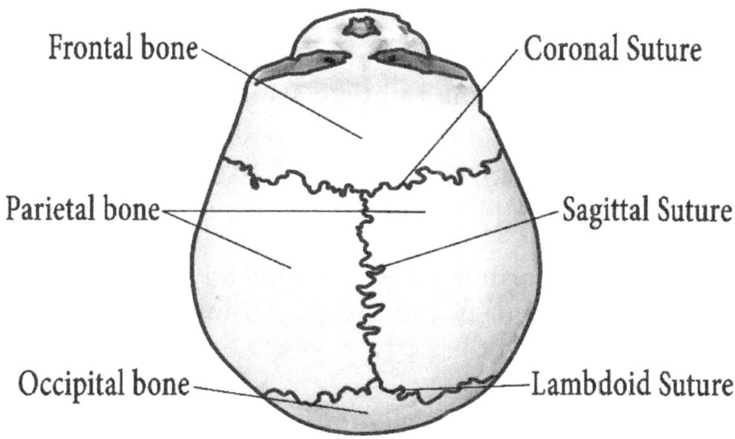

Figure 7. A skull (from above)

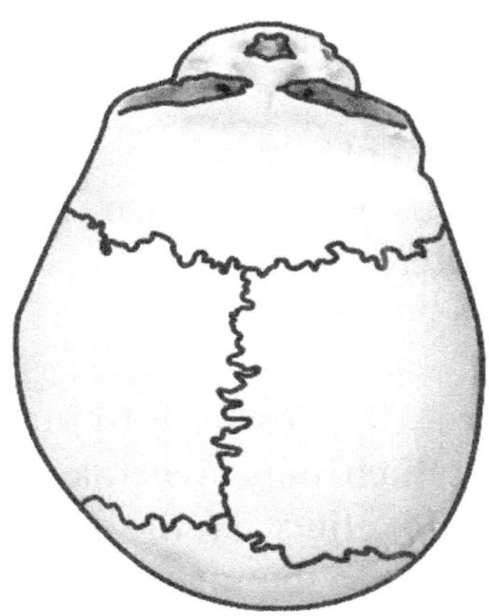

Figure 8. Torqued cranium (from above).

The words *torque* or *twists* imply a condition of *stress* which, in turn, suggests *restriction,* or *limitation.* And so it is. We can readily see that this cranium is rotated in such a manner that the right side of the head is further back relative to the left side. In a real person the right ear would be further back on the right side. The sutures must go with this torque and the *misalignment* of the cranial bones, one with the other, will impose a *stress* upon those sutures.

What a creaky garden gate you will have if the hinge is twisted. What, then, is the effect of those *torques* on our sutures? It is simply this:

There is a ***<u>limitation</u>*** *to* ***movement****.*

Instead of the peaks and troughs of our sine wave achieving *full amplitude* in both directions, there is *an impediment to the freedom of* ***movement*** caused solely by the abnormality of the alignment of the bones. It follows that the amplitude is altered and we may find ourselves with any one of countless departures from normal (maximum) such as we saw in Figures 3 and 4.

The engine, our source of *total function* of everything that is primary in making us what we are, is compromised and *cannot achieve its full potential* because the *casing* of the engine is warped.

And that, you will recall, goes back to birth, even in spite of other misfortunes which may overtake us on our journey through this life. The effect of the compromised level of function is to produce a panorama of what can best be described as *weaknesses* throughout the body and this is where much confusion can arise.

We (mostly) *appear* to be functioning normally. Perhaps more accurately, what we *consider* to be "normal". But, in effect, we are not functioning *optimally*. So, I repeat.

None of us knows what it is like to function optimally.

Or anywhere near it. Until we do something about the misaligned casing and its engine, that is. We have come to accept what is *normal* for ourselves as being *optimal*. It rarely is and the difference is frequently a chasm.

Chapter 8.

The Source. Lou Gehrig

Minds are like parachutes; they work best when open.
Lord Thomas Dewar

We continue to function variously, with weaknesses which *provide the basis* for the onset of a wide range of disorders. Let me give you a couple of examples.

Mary, aged 31, walks, nay, hobbles into the office, ashen faced, can't sit on the chair and tells her story. That morning she got up out of bed in the normal way and heads for the shower. All is going well until she steps out and bends down to pick up the towel which had fallen onto the floor. At that moment of bending, a severe shooting pain in her lower back sends her crashing to the floor. She calls for her husband, is eventually taken by ambulance to Emergency. Six months after the onset she appears in my office. Meantime she has been through various hands, had bed rest, traction, had seen two chiropractors, an acupuncturist and was now awaiting surgery. She was eating pain killers. Could I help?

In Mary's mind, naturally, she attributed this personal disaster to the innocent act of bending to pick up the towel, causing something "to go out". But, are we so feebly built that a simple act of bending – even with an element of twisting, or anything else – could be the cause of turning Mary's life around? After all, a towel is not exactly heavy either. What, then, lay behind this horrendous episode in her life?

Sure enough, the *act* of bending triggered off a chain of events that the body was unable to deal with. Of course, she had been having the odd twinge from time to time, and a couple of times she had to take time off work. But that wasn't even worth a mention, was it? The real problem was that Mary's *cranial, and neurological functional,* status had been increasingly producing a tension, or tightening, build up in the low back area, including misalignments of the vertebrae and pelvis. All of this had been proceeding *silently* – or more or less – without any awareness on Mary's part.

The important significance is that

its origin lay in the status of Mary's cranial mechanism,

and the increasing inability of a particular group of the body's structures to cope. There was a progressive inability of the muscle groups to assume a *fully relaxed* state, with the result that the *pre-existing tension* in the muscles of the back were easily triggered into that final spasm.

It was not Mary's low back locally (segmentally) that needed to be addressed, but the origin of *that pre-existing muscular tension,* her cranium. Yes, a long way from her low back, indeed. It was the *underlying* or *predisposing* weakness that had to be addressed and was the reason that the patient's symptoms were hanging on; they just couldn't get released until the *primary cause* had been attended to.

Then there was Michael, aged 44. He presented with a shoulder problem that had been troubling him on and off for many years. It had been originally dislocated on the football field, treated in Emergency and was now giving a lot of pain and with limited movement. The surgeons wanted to operate. But, as well as the shoulder, Michael had developed psoriasis, with itchy and bleeding patches mainly on his arms, elbows, legs, knees and trunk.

He didn't come to see me about the skin problems though. In his mind this one was for the dermatologist and for which he was already receiving treatment. Right, you're already ahead of me. Both problems had their origin at the cranial level and the psoriasis resolved too, in addition to the shoulder issue.

The *underlying functional weakness* had begun to show (symptoms) in terms of disturbance to the body's biochemistry as well as the muscular system. Hence the onset of the psoriasis. The lesson is, of course, that there is frequently a common connection between condition A and condition B (and C and D and so on), even though the nature of the symptoms, and the location of them, on the body may be far removed.

For example, a shoulder and a gall bladder; maybe a knee and a kidney; perhaps a balance problem and colitis. And not necessarily at the same time. The essential lesson that begins to emerge is that we need to begin to look *behind* the problem. We need to see the patient on a *total* or *global* basis. By that I mean we need to move our assessment away from a *fragmented* one in which "it" has to be targeted, to one in which he, or she, *in total*, has to be targeted.

In saying that, I'm aware that such an approach to healthcare is a million miles from most present-day practices. It is also as far removed from present day understandings as it can be. I believe it's time to turn our thinking around to a logical and effective one. It's time for a deeper understanding but, before moving on, it might be worth a pause to consider this one:

Lou Gehrig

Although a European, when I was teaching in the United States I recall frequently hearing reference to *Lou Gehrig's Disease* in response to my reference to *Motor Neurone Disease (MND)*. It is also referred to as *Amyotrophic lateral sclerosis (ALS).* Initially my question was: who was Lou Gehrig?

I now know, of course, that he was a baseball legend who needs no introduction on the American continent. Gehrig died in 1941, aged 37, from this crippling neurological disorder and for which, to this day, there is not a known successful medical response.
ALS attacks the motor neurons which are the nerve cells that control voluntary movements such as walking. There are two types of motor neurons, upper and lower. Upper motor neurons send messages from the brain to the spinal cord. Lower motor neurons carry the signals from the spinal cord to the muscles, telling them to move. Among the symptoms are progressive weakness of muscles, wasting of muscles, muscle twitching and developing difficulties in areas such as speaking, breathing and swallowing.

When researching the origins of the name given to this disease in the USA, I was struck by a report of an incident which occurred on June 29, 1934. In an exhibition game against Norfolk, VA, Gerhig was rendered unconscious by what is described as "a deliberate wild pitch" – presumably struck on the head - and was taken to hospital suffering from concussion.

It is reported that,

A few weeks later, he couldn't straighten up, said he had a "cold in his back," and left one game after the first inning. Gehrig would suffer similar bizarre attacks over the next few seasons, seemingly harbingers of his fatal disease. (www.answers.com)

I have been unable to find anywhere any suggestion that there may be a link between the concussion episode and the onset, soon after, of what seemed to be the first indications of the disease that was to follow. Nor does there appear to be any available record of details of the strike from the ball, such as the area of the head involved. Evidently such detail has been considered of no interest, or even relevance.

It is not being suggested that Gehrig's Disease is caused solely by injuries such as the one recorded in this case, and there are no doubt a number of possibilities, but there has to be more than a suggestion that Gehrig's fate was at least partially contributed to by the concussion incident.

It was also interesting that his low back episodes began to recur regularly very soon after this incident, and we have seen how low back problems are frequently related to the cranial status. The trauma to the head was clearly substantial and may well have resulted in significant dislocation to Gehrig's Primary Respiratory Mechanism.

At this time we will never know if, and to what degree, Gehrig's illness and career were impacted by the concussion incident. It may have been substantial.

Chapter 9.

The Laterality of Disease

It is better to understand a little than to misunderstand a lot.
Anatole France

We have seen how the weaknesses in the functioning of the organism, *irrespective of what the effects may be* – knee problem, colitis, rheumatoid, skin, sports and so on – often have their primary origin in *underlying* and *largely "silent"* weaknesses throughout the body. We have also seen that there are often, though not always, associated *trigger* factors involved. Mary's life was turned round for the worse by virtue of having stooped down to pick up a towel.

Was the act of stooping the real issue? No, it wasn't, even though she would no doubt have been fine if she hadn't made that movement. The point is that, if she hadn't made the movement that day, the real probability is that the same, or similar, reaction would have occurred at another time, another day, another year. It doesn't really matter. Further, even if the symptoms had more or less cleared by themselves, the underlying weakness would still have been there, all ready and primed to blow out again on another occasion.

The primary causal weakness must always be addressed.

Maximum functionality, or as near as one can get to it, must always be the objective, irrespective of the what, where or how the symptoms arose. To omit this *primary* level of the causative processes is, at best, to tinker around the edges of the disorder and, perhaps be helpful in some measure to the patient but, is still to leave the ***predisposing*** weakness in situ, only to leave the patient at risk of recurrence or, even for the problem to reinvent itself into another form - another "disorder".

Let me explain. The whole body is made up of two halves. By and large, the activity and status (over-contracted, over-relaxed) of structures on the left side are determined by the anatomical status of the left side of the cranium. Left side would include obvious areas such as left neck, left shoulder, left leg, left lung and left kidney. But, it would also include the spleen, located on the body's left side. Equally, right side would include the same obvious structures such as right leg, lung, kidney on that side and would also include, for example, the appendix, liver, gall bladder.

But, as we have seen with Henry, the alignments of craniums *on each side, left and right, are different.* So, therefore, will the effect of the *dural stress patterns* – the tensions, contractions - be different on each side of the body. When we bring together all the strands that make up *function*, including the all important nervous system, it means that the two sides of the body are working at different levels of function. It might be, for example, that in one person, the left side might be cranking along at, say, a 6.7 on our Richter scale of function, while the right might be at a, say, 5.2. As an interesting aside, we need to remember that some 80% of the nervous system originates within the cranium.

This anatomical difference between the two sides of any cranium is very common but, what does it mean? Well, it means simply that the right side in this person would be the "weaker" of the two. It is the side that is more likely to breakdown, more ***predisposed***, all other things being equal, throughout that person's lifetime. Maybe when you think back over your own lifetime you can think of having had more problems on one side than the other? Let me give you an example.

John, aged 61, arrived in the office complaining of persistent low back pain on the right side. This went back some 21 years. Here's a synopsis of his health history, so far as he could remember it and, so far as he believed these episodes were significant:

- Aged 4: tonsils removed.
- Aged 16: injury to right knee playing football
- Aged 21: right knee cartilage operation
- Aged 24: appendicitis operation
- Aged 26: left rib cage "injury" (didn't know how), followed by pain in left shoulder blade
- Aged 40: severe right side low back pain, right leg constantly cold, some right shoulder pain and right hand cold on and off
- Aged 42: ringing in the right ear - tinnitus
- Aged 55: through night bladder frequency, diagnosed as mild prostate

It will be seen that most of John's symptoms located to the right side of the body. That may, or may not, include the tonsil and bladder symptoms in addition, which are in the midline of the body and function neurologically from both sides, but all the indications, with the exception of the rib and shoulder blade injuries, are that the right side is the "weaker" side and the one more likely to breakdown.
So, we begin to understand what a knee, an appendix, a low back and an ear might have to do with each other. They are

all *victims* of the ONE flawed *over contracted* pattern on that side,

originating from the cranium.

In the world of the ***Bio Craniopathy***, the understanding is that, whatever the nature or location of disturbances on the one side of the body may be, there is a strong probability of a common factor between them. That common factor originates at the cranial - and associated structures - level and lays down the pattern of weaknesses from which these symptoms arise.

Let's take another example. Helen, aged 63, arrived in the office complaining she was falling apart. Her main complaints were headaches, increasing in number, and mostly above the left eye. She also referred to frequent bouts of palpitation of the heart and, in fact, she looked to be a very ill lady. A synopsis of her health history is as follows.

- Aged 17: first menstruation (much later than normal)
- Aged 23: diagnosis of "nervous breakdown" – continuation of these episodes intermittently for probably 20 years
- Aged 25: miscarriage
- Aged 26: operation for prolapsed womb
- Aged 42: diagnosis of angina
- Aged 48: menopausal
- Aged 52: gall stone surgery

In Helen's case, the "nervous breakdowns", angina and menopausal symptoms decidedly point to the left side, the gall stone episode to the right, and the others to either or both. From which we can reasonably conclude the probability that Helen's *weaker* side is on the left. And we now know why. Don't we? Of course, it's been determined at the cranial status and mostly, if not all, probably goes back to her birth.

And so we find ourselves moving back to the principles referred to in the first pages of this book. We are certainly made up of an array of diverse parts, but *they are all connected*. A few moments contemplation of the enormity and significance of this is worth a pause here.

Everything begins from the union of two cells and, from that, develops to bring about everything we now are, and do. This was not a haphazard sequence of events. This was intelligent and purposeful.

It follows that we refrain from meddling unnecessarily in a grand design that is infinitely beyond our comprehension in its design, function and purpose. Those areas are beyond the remit of mere mortals. Rather that we humble ourselves in recognition that our real knowledge of the miracle that is each of us is much further behind the learning curve than is supposed in many healthcare circles and will always remain so.

The real task is to acknowledge that the miracle has already been created, is potentially flawless and that the role of any professional in mediating dysfunction is to ***facilitate*** the restoration-to-normal process: to facilitate the organism's *innate wish* to function at its highest level. It's just crying out to do what it was designed to do. Which is to be free to *function normally.*

Chapter 10.

The Two Primary Lesions

The larger the island of knowledge, the longer the shoreline of wonder.
Ralph W. Sockman

The word *lesion* crops up frequently in the world of medicine. It's a non-specific word to describe any number of abnormalities or injuries to tissue or organ. Not surprisingly, there are many types of lesions and even sub types, but in straightforward terms they are essentially departures from normal. Or, the presence of an abnormality.

Thus, the dermatologist will refer to the skin lesion. A biopsy may then show that the skin lesion may be benign or malignant. The location of the abnormality may be the reason for the name such as, in the case of the neurologist, a central lesion will involve the brain or spinal cord, whereas a peripheral lesion will refer to nerves away from the spinal cord.

In my own case I was nurtured on the *osteopathic lesion*, a generic description which was mostly perceived to apply to anything to do with abnormalities of the body's structure and, particularly, to the skeleton. It also had its sub divisions, probably the most common of which was the *spinal lesion* which, as the name suggests, refers particularly to the bones of the spine. The vertebrae. The chiropractic community had their approximate equivalent, referred to as the *subluxation.*

The general consensus is that the joints of the vertebral column are subject to *mechanical* disturbance, or displacement. And there are some 89 articulations, including where ribs meet some of the vertebrae, and around which joints freely move in the spinal column.

In one sense, therefore, it seems reasonable to conclude that a column of bones, such as those that comprise the spine, are capable of being *mechanically* misaligned or displaced. And, indeed, abnormal positioning of vertebrae can be discerned radiographically, as well as by touch. So, *quod erat demonstrandum.* The vertebrae are capable of being displaced. And how else can that be, other than by trauma?

Within the professions the debate about the origins of the *spinal lesion* has gone on for many years and the most common of the reasons given, and universally agreed, is that of trauma. "The patient slipped on the wet floor, fell heavily and caused the *spinal lesion*". Which would seem to be entirely logical and, look there, the x-ray proves it.

But, if we had taken that X-ray *before* the patient fell, what would we have seen then? Would it have been normal? Or, would there have been evidence of a lesser lesion? Or, would that exact same radiographic evidence have been there in the first place and before the fall? In effect, are we correct in *assuming* that, because the patient was free of pain before the fall, she was therefore free of any *spinal lesion*?

We can't be sure, can we?

And so to the professional I ask this question: how many times have you examined a spine and found what you believed were spinal lesions, **but which had no associated symptoms on the part of the patient**?

This is where we need to revisit the cranium. Any cranium. For they will all carry some of the irregularities of the birthing process. They may well also carry additional trauma from the scars of living – fell down the stairs, banged the head on the car door, hit by the car mounting the pavement, it followed running the half marathon, lifting the turkey out of the oven. And so on.

We have already seen previously with Henry an example of how, and why, the two sides of the head are *asymmetrical.* One side may be lower than the other. Maybe twisted so that one side is further back than the other. Maybe even one side higher at the front and lower at the back than the other. These are all evidences of irregularities. They might be referred to as *cranial lesions.*

But, as we have seen, it doesn't end there. There are very important spin offs, one of which concerns the dural membrane. Remember that one? It's the membrane the attaches to the inside surface of the bones of the head and then runs down the length of the spinal cord as far as the tail bone.

Because of its attachment to the cranial bones - and let's not forget that these are in some degree of a *twist* – that twist, or torque, will be *imposed* on the ***dura***. The net result of which is that the ***dura mater*** assumes exactly the same equivalent torque, or twist, right down to the tail bone. Isn't that something? It's like follow-my-leader, the leader being the cranium.

The status of the dura matter is determined by the status of the cranial bones.

The stress pattern of the ***dura*** becomes a mirror image of that of the cranium. That torquing effect of the ***dura*** has a very important effect in that it results in a *tensioning* of this membrane. This membrane is no longer able to ***move freely***. It cannot assume the textbook status that it was designed for. Like its lord and master, the cranium, it is *lesioned.*

Next stop is the spine. All those vertebrae are now sitting there surrounded by a torqued and contracted ***dura mater*** and asking themselves the question, "Where do we fit in here? The only answer has to be: "No other option for us than to go to the most comfortable position we can find". The vertebrae react to this challenge by **all** assuming the most comfortable positions, in total, and which will allow them *to compensate* for the tension pattern imposed upon them by the ***dura***.

As a unit *each* vertebra will assume its best comfort zone *in conjunction with every one of its colleagues.* One moves this way. One moves another way and one moves yet another way. So that we have each vertebra assuming an abnormal position in its attempt to *compensate* for a *primary lesion* originating somewhere else – the cranium. And so, we have all of the vertebrae *in lesion*. Which they are. And these are the *secondary lesions.*

*The perceived vertebral lesions are mainly the **compensatory** lesions and seldom are primary lesions in themselves.*

Now, that will raise a few eyebrows among the professionals. The vertebral *sub lesions* are all the while striving their best to *accommodate* forces imposed upon them from the top. With the result, of course, that organ function, system function, neurological function, among others, associated with these structures are compromised.

Which brings us back again to this word *lesion.*

The balance of *function*, at all levels however, is essentially a two-way split. There are those that take place from the left side, and those that take place from the right. If, alone, we look at neurological function we are reminded that 80% of the nervous system originates in the brain. The remainder is from the spine. And where is the brain located other than within that casing we call the cranium?

The two-way split then refers to the impact the status of each half of the brain has on the other associated structures *on that same side of the body*. The stress pattern of the two halves of the *dura* will be different, as will be that of *all of the vertebrae* on both sides.

The level of nerve function on the two sides will be different, as will the level of function of the organs and systems supplies from each side, left or right.

One side is weaker than the other,

and is the one more susceptible to breakdown than the other. Bear in mind, however, that the "stronger" side is just that – stronger, but not necessarily *strong.*

Since the underlying balance and functionality of each side of the body is laid down at the cranial level the relative strengths and weaknesses will apply to

all structures, organs and systems on that side.

In the case of centrally located structures such as the bladder, in most cases the weaker side of that organ will still be on the overall weaker side of the body.

I refer to this phenomenon as

the Laterality of Disease/ Disorder.

As far as I'm aware, *this is the first time these phenomena had has been observed and recorded.* What then does this mean in practice? Well, firstly, we need to employ a bit of lateral thinking here. Contrary to current received wisdom, the ***Bio Craniopathic*** understanding now suggests that there is a *pre-existing weakness* in *all areas of function* and which is traceable back to the cranial status.

The presence, or otherwise, of symptoms is largely irrelevant.

It is this *underlying* weakness which primes the system for the onset of the symptoms some time up the line. This is the real – and unseen – culprit.

As we have seen, that weakness applies top to toe, and separately *each side of the body.* Which is why there may be a connection between, say, the bunion on the right toe and the right ear tinnitus that developed twenty years later. Both arose because of that right side weakness with that person. In effect the bunion fuse blew first, then the ear one. And who knows which fuse will blow next, *unless the cranial source of both problems is addressed first?*

We now come to the realisation that, in the ***Bio Craniopathic System,***

there are only two <u>primary</u> *lesions.*

There is the left sided lesion and,

there is the right sided lesion.

From each of these *lesions* spring the sub lesions such as the left knee *lesion*, almost certainly stemming from the primary *lesion* at the cranial level. Indeed, all the obvious structures on each side will almost certainly arise from the *primary lesion* on the same side. The right shoulder, the right side sciatica, the right hip, the right nostril, the right lung, the right kidney are all obviously on that one side.

RIGHT SIDE LESION

Some more central organs also relate to the right side, such as liver, gall bladder, duodenum and the digestive function of the pancreas. Associated with these structures would be disorders such as:

bloating, gall stones, some indigestions, constipation, ileocecal valve (appendix) problems and cholesterol issues.

LEFT SIDE LESION

On the left side, in addition to the obvious structures there, we would find the heart, of course, the spleen, the main body of the stomach (the fundus) and its hiatal valve which joins up with the tracheal tube.

These left side structures are involved in an interesting range of disorders. One of these is that the hormonal component of the pancreas functions from the left, rather than the right, side as for its digestive function. Thus, diabetes relates to the left side ***Bio Craniopathic*** *lesion*.

Also, from the left side we find a range of cardiac disorders, including angina. Other common maladies relating to the left side would include some anaemias, hiatal hernias, reflux, some anxieties, rheumatoid arthritis, (even though the *symptoms* of this are often bi-lateral), hyperactivity, some cases of overweight, especially in females and related to fluid retention associated with hormonal imbalances.

Alcoholism has a decided left side input, wherein the sufferer finds that the imperative is to feel *relaxed*, at ease within, and the overwhelming need can be satisfied from the relaxing effect of alcohol. Hence the growing dependency on it. The same can be said of the heavy smoker and, again, for the same reason: the need to satisfy the body's craving to be *relaxed*.

Within this framework we can also include the nail biter, generally regarded as an anti-social and undesirable habit but, in reality, is a practice which has the effect of indirectly releasing cranial restriction and tension in the area of the jaw – the tempero-mandibular joint (TMJ). Do you ever wonder why the persons labelled "of nervous disposition" talk so much? I suspect the constant ***movement*** of that TMJ provides a measure of release for which the *overcontracted* system is crying out.

On this basis, of course, the *act* of eating will have a similar effect and so will not only provide the required nutrition, but will provide the pleasurable *relaxing* effect as part of the process. Little wonder we all enjoy eating so much.

The left side, particularly, is a fascinating one. It is our driving, our achieving, one. The left side dominant people are never happier than when engaged in ***movement***. That ***movement*** is expressed in many ways such as impatience, (shifting from one foot to the other, tapping the fingers on the desk, and so on). I suspect that it is the dominant side in many of our captains of industry, and so there are both positive and negative characteristics.

It should be understood that, in none of the disorders listed above, is it suggested that the ***Bio Craniopathic System*** lesion is the only factor involved in the names listed and it is always recommended that sufferers from any of those listed disorders, and others, should seek advice from their chosen professional advisers. It has been found, however, that the lateralities, left or right, are as I've indicated.

It should also be emphasised that none of us is dominantly weak *solely* on one side or the other. My own estimate is that some 70% of us are *significantly dominant* on one side, left or right, and the remainder show little difference on susceptibility between the two sides.

The important point, however, is that few of us are firing on all cylinders on both sides but with a majority more so on one side or the other.

By now it will be appreciated that the goal becomes one of *relaxation*. That is the state that the body longs for innately, instinctively, intuitively. The state of *relaxation* embraces the concepts of openness, release, freedom from restraint. It is the natural order. When did you ever hear anyone say, "Just can't wait to go on vacation to get *contracted*"?

Chapter 11.

Cranial Anatomical Flexion

Nothing endures but change.
Heraclitus

It will be appreciated by this time that the ***Bio Craniopathic System*** derives from a unique philosophical base, even within all of the cranial based disciplines. And it is those same understandings that result in its treatment protocol,

which is exactly the same for each patient, irrespective of the nature of the presenting disorder.

Remarkable, isn't it? So let me explain.

It will be apparent now that most illnesses/disorders have their *primary* origin in layers of weaknesses laid down at birth (and before), and which will follow us throughout life. I've referred to this as the *predisposing* level in the causation processes and relates to weaknesses in *any* of the body's systems caused primarily by the abnormality of the cranial system. Simply put, each of us operates at a level of function ***which is below that which is possible and for which we were designed.***

In order to move from the present level of function towards the optimum one possible it is essential that the anatomical status of the cranial system *in total* (and *dura* etc) be changed to a specific status which I have designated as one of

Anatomical Flexion.

This is a technical term which requires no further elaboration here. It is, however, not any part of any other discipline that I am aware of, and is therefore unique to the ***Bio Craniopathic System***. It is suffice to think of it as the objective in which the patient's level of function is moved progressively from, say, a level 4.6 or 6.2 or 7.1 on our Richter scale to as near to the maximum possible for each patient – theoretically, say, level 10.

You will note that we are not referring to symptoms, or the names of disorders – perhaps back pain, cerebral palsy, torn knee cartilage, varicose ulcer, tinnitus, colitis and so on – all of which will carry ***a predisposing burden of functional weakness***. Why, then, address the *local,* or symptomatic area (knee, ulcer and so on) when the underlying ***primary*** issue was the reason for the breakdown in the first place?

Will that alone be enough to resolve the problem? Let me answer that by asking another question. Was not the body designed to be ***self-healing****?* Of course, it was, and, ***even in the presence of the most serious disorders***, it is striving for all its worth for normality – health. It is merely crying out to be "released" to achieve that objective.

But what about all those disorders brought about by the myriads of injuries that beset us? The heavy tackle on the football field? The slip on the ice? The whiplash? The fall from the horse? On the face of it there appears to be a direct connection between the incident and the injury.

And there is no denying it.

The question arises, however, as to the extent to which there was a ***predisposing weakness*** in the first place and which was primary in contributing to the trauma in question. The sporting world is awash with players and athletes suffering from injuries which fall into this category and, in my experience, resolve quickly and more fully if addressed by ***Bio Craniopathy***.

Obvious exceptions to this would be where there had been serious and major trauma. Most trauma, however, is at a much lower level than this and usually requires little more than to have the ***predisposing*** weaknesses addressed, whether it be the hamstrings, the shoulder, the wrist, the knee, the neck and so on.

So what might the patient expect in the hands of the skilled ***Bio Craniopathic*** practitioner? Broadly speaking the expectation level of most patients falls into one of two categories:

1. Get rid of this pain (or whatever) as soon as possible, OR
2. Help me achieve my best possible health level.

The big difference between the two is that the former is almost entirely ***symptom driven***. The red flag is up; the warning signals are there that all is not well, maybe seriously so. Time to do something. The latter may begin the same way and then progress to another level.

Most of us fall into category 1 for a variety of reasons, the main one being that our current understandings are that *there is not a problem unless recognisable/ identifiable symptoms are present.* All of which is very understandable.

The general perception is that the job is done when the symptoms are gone – or nearly so.

As will now be appreciated, ***Bio Craniopathy*** addresses ***only*** the deeper level of the causative processes and which are ***total*** within the body and not ***local*** (knee, gall bladder, skin and so on). It is the totality of the disorder which has ***predisposed*** to the local breakdown and is therefore what must be addressed. The imperative is to change the weakness at a level hitherto beyond our knowledge and understandings.

The treatment protocol of ***Bio Craniopathy*** is a process of taking the flawed status of the patient, and which underpins the dysfunction, and progressively moves that anatomical status to an objective of *openness*, or *release*, which then in turn allows ALL of the body's structures and systems to maximise. It is a process of facilitating the body to ***correct and heal itself***.

It is important to understand that the resolution of the symptoms is effectively an *unravelling* process. It's like pealing the layers off an onion. For the most part the weaknesses being addressed and corrected have been there for 20 years in the twenty-year-old; for 40 years in the forty-year-old; for 70 years in the seventy-year-old. Further, the extent, or depth, of the dysfunction will vary enormously from one person to another.

For that reason the twenty-year-old may be dysfunctionally in a weaker state than the seventy-year-old. Age is not the only determinant. The ***Bio Craniopathic System*** is definitely *not* a patch-up approach directed at some localised area. It is the reason why *diseases/ disorders*, as such are *NOT treated*. It is the whole person that is *treated*, irrespective of the names we are used to appending to the disorder – psoriasis, tumour, diabetes, sciatica, rib, rheumatoid and so on.

In practice, however, most of us are content to settle for *unravelling* the process to the point of being free of symptoms. And that is progress. That is improved functionality, whether it be an apparently innocuous low back pain or perhaps an organ or system disturbance. For those, however, who are seeking something more than merely the relief of symptoms and to maximise their level of function, it will be understood that there is a marked difference between being more or less symptom free on the one hand, and performing to the maximum extent, on the other. The latter is about ***wellbeing***. It is about energy levels; about feeling focused; about feeling co-ordinated; about clarity of thought; about being at ease with oneself; about a feeling of wholeness and, in all probability, even about the life span itself. And so much more and, not least, being less susceptible to health breakdowns as the years go by.

The present level of dysfunction with all of us will have been impacted from many sources – nutritional, cultural, heredity, lifestyle, family to name a few. In some cases one or more of these external factors may be very significant and, if possible, require to be addressed. Irrespective of any other factors, however, I am clear in my mind that the issue of *functionality* as described in this book will almost always be the primary one to be addressed for a very wide range of people.

Part 2

The Master System

I shall be telling this with a sigh
Somewhere ages and ages hence;
Two roads diverged in a wood, and I --
I took the one less traveled by,
And that has made all the difference.

Robert Frost

Chapter 12.

The Body's Master System

Some circumstantial evidence is very strong, as when you find a trout in the milk.
Thoreau

We are well used to references to the various systems which go to make up the totality of function in the body. Even these, in turn, are subject to differing classifications and one definition of bodily systems is that they are the ***largest elements of the human body that have critical functions.***

On that basis the following ten groupings may be considered to constitute general acceptance of what goes to make us what we are:

1. **Circulatory system**: pumping blood to and from the body and lungs.
2. **Lymphatic system**: structures involved in the transfer of lymph between tissues and the blood stream.
3. **Musculoskeletal system**: movement with muscles and involving the human skeleton.
4. **Nervous system**: collecting, transferring and processing information between the brain, spinal cord and nerves.
5. **Reproductive system**: the sex organs.

6. **Urinary system**: kidneys, ureters, bladder and urethra.
7. **Respiratory system**: the pharynx, larynx, trachea, bronchi, lungs, and diaphragm.
8. **Endocrine system**: the hormonal system including such structures as the hypothalamus, pituitary gland, pineal gland, thyroid, parathyroids, and adrenal glands.
9. **Digestive system**: the digestive processes including salivary glands, oesophagus, stomach, liver, gallbladder, pancreas, intestines.
10. **Integumentary system**: skin, hair and nails.

Did you spot what's missing here? There is something very important missing.

By this time it will be apparent that, *behind the functioning of every one of the above systems,* there is what might be called a ***Master System***.

Disorders of, say, the liver – part of the digestive system – will often be traceable back to a ***predisposing*** dysfunction originating at the cranial level.

Equally, a respiratory issue – say asthma – is very likely to have its roots in a dysfunction at the cranial level.

Then again, the irregular menstruation of the young female involving the endocrine (hormonal) system, has in all likelihood its origins in cranial dysfunction.

And so on. In effect there is not one of the above listed systems that is not ***primarily dependent*** for its integrity and full function on the cranial mechanism. So, here's the dilemma.

The present state of knowledge in the world of medicine <u>doesn't even</u> <u>know</u> of the existence of movement of the cranial structures.

Which means that any medical mediation in any of the above systems is taking place in the absence of any awareness of the *dependency* of all of them on a ***higher*** system – the motor system which is the driving force upon which most function relies.

In effect, the systems of the body, as are presently known and referred to, are subservient to a hitherto unrecognised system which is the ***Master System***. The others are *entirely dependent* upon this ***System*** and, even if requiring to be addressed separately at times, there will almost always be the need to address the ***Master System***. This ***System***, previously unrecognised, and therefore without a name, will logically *<u>take precedence</u> over all other Systems.*

Man's ingenuity has evolved and developed a vast range of protocols to address disorders of the *dependent* systems. Some are life saving. Some are helpful. Some are useless. Some are even dangerous.

But wouldn't it be so much more beneficial if the *Controller* of all other Systems, were taken into account? We might just ponder how much an intervention at this level might change the dynamics in favour of the patient, not to mention the oft struggling physician or practitioner. Indeed, it might just eliminate, or at the very least reduce, the need for many other interventions. After all, we keep coming back to it. Were we not designed to self-heal, from within, given the *openness*, the balance, the body is crying out for?

If, therefore, this newly recognised ***Master System*** is to take its rightful place as the body's major System there then needs to be a reappraisal of certain of the other Systems. The new ***Master System***, being the source of *movement* in all other Systems – and therefore *function* - is mainly constituted from component parts of the present ***Nervous System*** and ***Musculoskeletal System***.

The ***Nervous System*** is extremely complex and is made up of many parts, but it is generally recognised to consist of two main *Systems*. There is firstly the ***Central Nervous System (CNS)*** consisting of the brain and the spinal cord, and then the ***Peripheral Nervous System (PNS)***, consisting of the nerve cells and the *wiring* between them.

The ***Musculoskeletal System*** consists of the two components, *muscular* and *skeletal*, and are often linked together simply because the body's muscles activate the skeleton. In the new knowledge of the *existence* of the *controller* of all Systems, the ***Master System***, it seems more proper to assign the ***whole of the Nervous System*** to constituting a ***part*** of the *Master System* rather than to considering it as one of the *dependent* System. So to the ***Nervous System*** we extend our congratulations on your promotion.

However, to the ***Musculoskeletal System*** we must downgrade you even further and separate the two components. The muscular component goes its separate way and remains one of the *dependent* Systems. The ***skeletal*** component is promoted to become a ***part*** of the ***Master System***. It, too, has two parts known as the ***axial skeleton*** and comprises all 29 bones of the cranium, including the hyoid and bones of the inner ear, the ribs and the whole of the vertebral bones. The second part is known as the ***appendicular skeleton*** and consists of some 126 bones connected directly or indirectly to the ***axial skeleton***. The

skeletal component attaches anatomically *directly* to the cranium – ***movement*** – at the first spinal vertebra.

The other extremely important component of the *Master System* is the one foreshadowed by Dr Sutherland and which he called the *Reciprocal Tension Membrane* and referred to the outer of the three membranes which cover the brain and spinal cord and also attach to some of the bones of the cranium and vertebral column. This is, of course, the ***Dura mater,*** the great connector between the cranium and spinal cord/ vertebrae.

In summary the ***Master System*** would comprise:

1. The Cranium
2. The Central Nervous System (CNS)
3. The Skeleton
4. The Dura mater

The ***Musculoskeletal System*** is replaced by the ***Muscular System*** while the previously listed ***Nervous System*** becomes a part of the new ***Master System***.

But all of this only if you know of the *existence* of the ***Master System*** which you, dear reader, are privy to.

Chapter 13.

The Psychosomatic Dimension

Take rest; a field that has rested gives a bountiful crop.
Ovid

Another question then arises: to what extent are disorders of the *mind* and disorders of the physical – the soma – connected? Or not connected? Is there an overlap or, are they separate *compartments*?

The term *psychosomatic* is defined as:

of, relating to, involving, or concerned with bodily symptoms caused by mental or emotional disturbance. (Merriam-Webster.com).

The term itself suggests the causative process as being one where the psyche (mind) is a cause of certain disorders of the soma (physical). And there can be few of us who have not witnessed a clear connection between events such as shock, fear or anxiety, affecting an individual – perhaps as close as ourselves – and the onset of a physical disorder.

There is then that group of disorders which may appear to be located in the *mind* compartment only, without any, or little, apparent connection to a physical disorder – bi-polar, schizoid, depression, dementia and so on. The treatment plans for this category are mainly in the area of medication or psychotherapy or both.

Some physical diseases are believed to be particularly prone to being triggered, or aggravated, by mental factors such as stress and anxiety. Examples would be high blood pressure, psoriasis, eczema, gastric ulcers, and heart disease. It is believed that the physical symptoms, (rash, palpitation, blood pressure), can be affected from the psychological source. However, this is generally acknowledged as being difficult to prove.

The mechanisms behind the psychosomatic phenomenon are still speculative though one suggestion, for example, is that physical symptoms arise from an 'overdrive' of nerve impulses from the brain to various parts of the body, and to adrenaline being released into the bloodstream in the presence of anxiety. So we have some common ground here – the brain. And we know it resides within the cranium. And the brain is, of course, subject to ***movement***. We are back to the ***Master System***.

Why, then, is there such a divergence of reactions between people to these disparate external influences to which we are all subject? Why do some sit in apparent oblivion when the plane hits the turbulence while others assume the near panic mode? Why do some people externalise symptoms such as eczema in the days, or weeks, before an important event such as the final interview for the job, while others take it in their stride?

I recall a patient who confessed to me that she had been a "worrier" all her life, even when there was no reason for her to worry about anything. "Why am I like this?" she asked. "My husband can't understand me". Then why do some strive to avoid any situation which they recognise as having the potential to produce stress, anxiety and which, in turn, they fear will cause the blood pressure to rise? Are these, and like, circumstances the result of intrinsic personality features? Something that is there as part of the inheritance from birth? Something one is stuck with and has to learn to live with?

This is a complex and little understood area of our *being-ness* and there are clearly many considerations and influences in determining who and what each of us is. Included in this, for example, would be familial background, cultural exposure, education, religious background and so on. I am not, therefore, going to attempt to outdo Hegel, Aristotle or any of the other great minds who have addressed these, and other, aspects of the Great Questions.

Nevertheless, in the early stages of the development of ***Bio Craniopathy*** I did begin to notice that changes to the ***Master System***, mostly applied for physical type disorders, were often bringing about gratifying changes in the *personality/ psychological* field as a kind of off-shoot to the main business at hand – physical disorders. The possible causative mechanisms may have been mainly, even solely, of psychological origin. It was impossible to tell. It was also impossible to determine if the results were due to physiological changes only – improved hormone function, better blood supply (and therefore nutrition), etc.

Let's lay it out simply with one of a number of cases.

Trevor, 55 years old, presented with a medical diagnosis of prostate enlargement and low back pains, which were his chief complaints. He had a history of low back problems including surgery to the first and second lumbar vertebrae. He also had had an episode of left kidney stones (calculus) when 42 for which he was hospitalised and was currently on medication for high blood pressure.

The patient duly received ***Bio Craniopathic*** treatment which was successful for all his presenting symptoms, including the blood pressure, for which he elected to progressively reduce his medication in association with his own physician.

After three or four visits, however, Trevor, who by this time had developed a heart warming smile, in contrast to earlier visits, announced, "Feeling great. My wife says she can live with me now". (I think, *so now he tells me?*). I reply, "Oh, were there problems at home?" "Yes," he replied, "for most of my life I've been a bit of a recluse. Didn't want to go out into company. Always had this fear thing. Afraid of looking foolish. I never liked being away from home and I'd easily fly into a rage, often over very simple things and then I'm full of apologies for embarrassing people. Couldn't help myself". These are not the words verbatim but are pretty close to our actual conversation.

Trevor went on to relate what were to him the dramatic changes in his demeanour and even personality following his treatments. He felt relaxed within himself to a degree never before experienced. His head was clear. He had more energy. He and his wife had booked a holiday together, the first since their honeymoon. He wanted – yes, actually wanted – to meet with people.

The question I asked myself from this, and other, encounters was: were these behavioural features previously present as a result of just not feeling well physically? Even going back all those years? Were they the result of an inner frustration at his inability to escape from the straightjacket into which he seemed to be locked physically? Were the psychological factors effectively *a reaction to* the physical disorders?

Or was it the other way around? Were the personality/ psychological symptoms wholly, or partly, responsible for the physical symptoms? What comes first, the chicken or the egg?

Then there was the group of disorders which are believed to "reside" in the realm of the psychological sphere and where symptoms were identified as of psychological *in origin.* These would include anxiety, depression, post-traumatic stress, panic attacks, bipolar, insomnia, schizophrenia and even disorders commonly associated with children such as ADHD.

Many of these are believed to have recognizable, and associated, chemical abnormalities. For example, depression and anxiety are believed to be caused by chemical changes in the brain. In these disorders, chemicals called 'neurotransmitters', which are manufactured and released in the brain, become diminished in availability. The main neurotransmitters involved with psychological problems are Serotonin (5HT), Norepinephrine (Noradrenalin) and Dopamine. All have different effects but without the correct levels of these chemicals there is emotional and psychological instability.

It began to progressively dawn on me that the vast majority of both so-called psychological and psychosomatic disorders had their origin in the ***left side Master System lesion***. I began to notice that a number of characteristics exhibited by those around us had their commonality on the left side. Among these would be:

1. Those who are unable to sit, or stand, still for any length of time – assuming there is no other physical reason for it.
2. The grinder of the teeth during sleep.

3. The finger tapper.
4. The nail biter.
5. The short tempered – they can't absorb stress, are impatient (can't wait for an answer or outcome: it means waiting)
6. The impatient – as in 5.
7. The aggressive type.
8. The big ego type.
9. The shy, the diffident, the blusher, including the menopausal flashing.
10. The avoider of controversy.

These virtual non-symptoms are usually dealt with by the person in one of two ways. The first, such as the shy person, is by deliberately refraining, where possible, from a circumstance which might precipitate any *discomfort* – avoidance, steering clear. The other is dealt with, mostly subconsciously, by ***movement***. We have seen how, and why, the underlying and therefore predisposing, status of dysfunction is one of *contraction.* This state is not always accompanied by clearly defined symptoms, of course, but is recognized by the body's innate intelligence as being in need of release.

Movement, such as drumming the fingers on the desk, will provide *temporary* respite and release for the organism.

The innate intelligence of the body knows best what it needs and that is to be as free as possible to function. And here I will add to that my own theory. I confess it can be no more than that.

The left side of the body comes within the remit of the left side ***Master System***. Apart from the obvious structures such as left shoulder, arm, leg and so on, there would be left kidney, left lung, spleen and, importantly, the hormonal function of the pancreas (diabetes). The left side lesion will also include the cardiac system, that absolutely critical system to sustaining the body's essential processes. If that system is recognized by the innate intelligence as being *under threat*, the result will be a rush, subconsciously, to protect it in whatever way possible and however temporary. Hence the resort to *movement*. In the case of the shy person, the mechanism appears to be simply one of being non-confrontational.

It is also very possible, even probable, that dysfunction at the cranial level will result in phenomena such as the chemical changes suggested by some researchers. In other words, the chemical changes are an *effect* rather than a *cause*. My own conclusion, however, has been that, irrespective of whatever *precipitating* events may be involved in triggering the mind > body psychosomatic response – shock, anxiety, fear and so on – the primary consideration is most often the ***somatico-psyche*** one, in which the soma, the physical, in the form of the ***Master System*** is a primary area requiring to be addressed. In my experience, if such an approach is followed the *predisposition to reaction from the external influences* is transformed.

If accepted, the implications of this theory within society could be substantial. My mind turns to the criminal population and prison services, for example. My understanding is that within that population there is a much greater proportion of inmates with attributable psychological disturbance than is to be found in the general population. No surprises there. One can only speculate on the impact the application of ***Bio Craniopathic*** principles would have in this area, both socially and economically.

Drug abuse, again common within the prison population, but extends even wider, relates frequently to the left side lesion and this is not surprising when one considers that it is an *instrument* for inducing what the body is always crying out for – relaxation, release. The abuser has found a source that fulfills that need and has progressively built a reliance on it to such a degree that dependency finally ensues.

I should add that there is no suggestion that these, and other, issues are entirely resultant from the left side ***Master System*** lesion status. They are merely suggested as worthy of relevance and exploration, and arise from my own observation and experience, however limited that has been.

Chapter 14.

Nutrition, Extrinsic/ Intrinsic

The first law of dietetics seems to be if it tastes good, it's bad for you.
Isaac Asimov

The health, or otherwise, of any of the cells in the body depend upon many factors, not least of which would be the nutrition taken into the organism. The food chain is itself subject to a wide variety of social and environmental influences such as soil quality, rainfall patterns, crop rotation, agricultural chemicals, food processing and other factors. Both quantitatively and qualitatively there are wide variations in the nutritional intake of individuals, even within the same household for that matter.

Broadly speaking the issue of what we take into our bodies embraces that area of *extrinsic nutrition*, a subject upon which volumes have been written, often with conflicting opinions and I'm not proposing to add further to this ongoing debate.

There is, however, another level to the subject of nutrition which is at least as important to the wellbeing of the organism, but about which I'm unaware of little recognition, let alone information, being available on it. I'm here referring to the subject of *intrinsic nutrition*. It is quite possible to ingest the most wonderful food in the world – whatever that may be – and yet be undernourished. Once the food is taken into the body there is then another task in hand which is to digest, extract, assimilate and distribute those nutrients. If any of these tasks is *dysfunctioning* it follows that there will be a shortfall in satisfying the body's needs.

The major source of nutrition to the cells is by means of the blood supply carrying elements such as glucose, amino acids, fats, oxygen, enzymes and mineral salts – all essential to cellular metabolism. Cellular health is also dependent upon the efficient removal of waste products such as urea, uric acid, creatinine, lactic acid and carbon dioxide. There must therefore be an *unimpeded* flow of nutrition *to,* and elimination *from,* the cell.

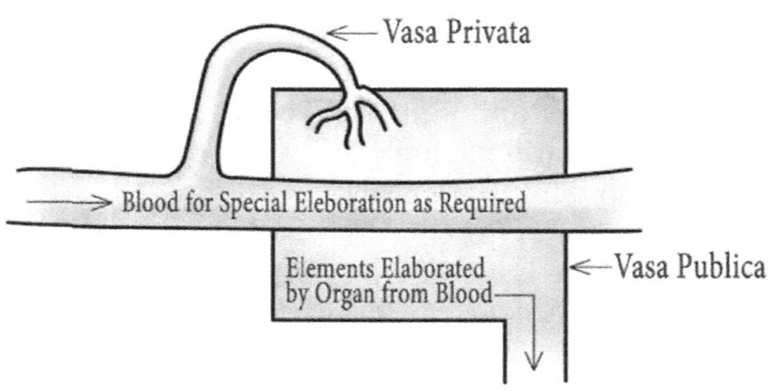

Fig. 9

Let's consider a simple example of how this might affect an organ in the body - any organ which might be, say, a liver or a kidney. In Figure 9, we can see, from the left, the blood supply arriving at the organ (Vasa Privata), supplying the nutrition *to the cells of the organ*, thus supporting their wellbeing needs. The organ's cells, of course, then have the task of converting that nutrition into the materials for which those cells were designed.

These materials, in turn, are then transported *from the organ's* cells (Vasa Publica) to other structures in order to allow them, in turn, to complete their function and *which were not necessarily in the extrinsic food chain.*

What if, now, we find there is an inherent weakness in the mechanism? Suppose the blood vessels supplying the nutrients to the cells are lesioned, *contracted*, by virtue of the nerve function controlling the muscular walls of the conveying mechanism, the blood vessels, being in lesion (***Master System***) the result will be less blood flow and therefore diminished nutrition *to* the cells of the organ.

The *purpose* for which the cells of the organ were designed will then be affected in two ways:

1. There will be inadequate nutrition available from which to convert to the materials for which the cells of that organ were designed to elaborate and distribute. Their *function* is compromised.

2. If there is a similar, malfunction of the nerve supply controlling the blood vessels *from* the organ to its target structures, there may well be another problem. The vessels carrying the newly elaborated materials may be *contracted*. The result is that the diameter of the blood vessel is *narrowed* and the *quantity* of manufactured material available for distribution is diminished. This amounts to localised malnutrition, *intrinsically caused.*

The mechanism underpinning this flawed situation is the ***Master System***. Cellular health must be nutritionally based and changes from normal health to abnormal must contain at least elements of what might best be called *malnutrition*, whether it be of *extrinsic* or *intrinsic* origin, or both. My own belief is that this is a much-neglected area of our understandings in our search for answers to a wide range of illnesses and will have particular relevance where pathological changes are present, whether that be simple inflammation or other pathological changes, right up to tumour formation.

Again, this is not to say that, by addressing the ***Master System*** all will be healed, but it is here suggested, and based on clinical experience, that the much-neglected *intrinsic nutritional factor* is of considerable significance and plays a much greater role in the causation processes than is generally appreciated. Not surprising really, when few are aware of the existence of the mechanism involved.

Chapter 15.

Diagnosis

Still round the corner there may wait,
A new road or a secret gate.
JRR Tolkien

Medical diagnosis has become an industry. Part of this is due to the advances in technology and part due to the perceived need to discern an abnormality of something, somewhere, which may be relative to the patient's disorder. Patients demand a name. Doctors are required to follow particular protocols for various symptoms. Beneficiaries include the drug companies and the chain of supporting individuals, research organizations, advocacy groups, insurance industry and many more. The list goes on.

Over-diagnosis therefore becomes increasingly common and the pressure is on the front-line physician, for example, to prescribe some medication for the patient, whether he believes it to be appropriate or not. The same applies to patient insistence for expanded investigation, whether or not such a course is believed to be necessary.

The criterion for diagnosis continues to change. Over the years the ubiquitous cholesterol diagnosis has continued to change. A routine blood pressure check for an apparently unrelated disorder can result in a lifetime of prescription medication. All manner of tissue changes from minor to major can now be detected with the use of increasingly sophisticated technology. The result is that we can overnight migrate from normality to being "at risk" and finding ourselves on to a course of any of a plethora of "preventative" measures, including medication.

It is enough, of course, that there should be *real* and *significant* disorders without there being an ever-increasing number of fanciful ones. In an article in the British Medical Journal (*BMJ* 2002;324:886-891 (13 April)) the authors commented on the practice of drug companies *disease mongering* including .... *turning ordinary ailments into medical problems, seeing mild symptoms as serious, treating personal problems as medical, seeing risks as diseases, and framing prevalence estimates to maximise potential markets.*

We are, however, a disease orientated society in contradistinction to many of the great civilisations of the past where much greater emphasis was placed on *wellbeing*. Almost all our actions in relation to personal health are precipitated by the presence of *symptoms*. Or, as referred to, by being virtually stampeded by reckless and often subtle marketing *without* the presence of symptoms.

From a diagnostic perspective it is readily understandable that symptoms are indicators that something is awry. They may present in an instant, such as the fall from the slip on the floor, or slowly and perhaps insidiously over a time frame or, perhaps intermittently. They may be severe or barely recognisable or anywhere in between. They may require instant help, professionally or self-administered or may apparently be self-resolving.

For the most part, and by far, they are the measurement by which we make judgements as to whether we are *healthy* or *functioning normally.* They are the *symptoms,* as determined by the patient and from which usually flow the *diagnosis* subjectively or professionally. In this scenario the *causative* factors assume some significance. They may be obvious – "I fell down the stairs…." or much less so – "this intermittent nausea has been building up for a year or so…."

Nevertheless, there is commonly an assumption that the patient's disorder *began* around the time of the first awareness of *symptoms* appearing and that, by implication, all was well beforehand. And there are indeed often a host of potential factors which may have played some part in both the development, and onset, of a particular disorder. Obvious examples would be dietary indiscretions, years of suppressive medication for previous minor illnesses, a few heavy falls in the ski slopes, over fondness for alcohol and/ or tobacco. And so on. There are, however, broadly two major determinants in the *causative* processes which in turn play into the *diagnostic* outcome.

Vertical (or Snapshot) Assessments

The first of these is the one alluded to above and which may be referred to as the *Vertical Assessment.* They are functional or pathological deviations *at any given moment in time* and are usually *symptomatically* driven. They are also usually *segmentally* orientated by which is meant that the focal area of the symptoms becomes the main pursuit. This would be particularly true, for example, in disturbances such as carpel tunnel syndrome, duodenal ulcer, herpes zoster, etc. It would also apply in systemic disorders such as rheumatoid, acne, fibromyalgia, multiple sclerosis etc, where the *symptoms* may be widespread but the *cause* is believed to be linked to perhaps one system as in the endocrine one.

It is essentially a reading at any given moment in time, and is generally one of the status of the patient at that moment, whether generated from a symptom picture or from a diagnostic investigation. The procedures may include areas such as radiography, various scans, laparoscopies, breast screening, blood tests, allergy testing and similar procedures, some of which are intrusive and/or highly invasive.

The diagnostic outcome is therefore similarly localized, or *segmental,* and seeks to identify the area of dysfunction or tissue abnormality accordingly. The diarrhoea (the symptom) may be diagnosed as ulcerative colitis (the diagnosis following investigative procedures), leading to the determination of the treatment protocol *for that disorder at that moment.*

In the absence of any other symptoms the story usually ends there apart from some other possible peripheral findings that may emerge – low red cell count, low potassium levels and so on. There is not, however, any sense that the colitis may just be part of a larger issue in which the colitis "fuse" has blown segmentally and that it may be a signal that a hole has appeared in the gentleman's shirt but that the real cause lay in the poor weave of the cloth in the first place, and not just from normal wear and tear. We can't, of course, replace the weave of our bodies but we can do even better. We can improve the inherent level of our co-ordinated functionality *so that the susceptibility to breakdown, anywhere, is vastly improved.* And even when localized breakdown has occurred the weakness underpinning it is changed for the better and forever.

Horizontal Assessment

In this area we have the hitherto unrecognised functional weaknesses laid down at birth and before.

It is a continuum over our lifetimes.

It is laid down at birth and before and will govern the *level* at which every system, every organ, every cell will function. It will be paramount in determining the level at which the co-ordination processes of the total organism will perform and therefore the degree to which the susceptibility to breakdown will take place. The level of health and wellbeing.

This is the *Horizontal Assessment* of our functionality. It will not be a constant throughout our lifetimes. It will not be a constant even from day to day, hour to hour and minute to minute. It will be subject to the vagaries of living such as stress, age, nutritional variations, climate, environment and others but there will nevertheless be a *mean* level at which function will be present *and which will be critical and basic in determining our predisposition to most disorders and many injuries.*

It follows that, even in the presence of a disorder, including those where pathology is present, it is a given that the *predisposition* is addressed in almost all cases, irrespective of what other protocols are deemed necessary or desirable.

This scenario may be represented as follows:

BIRTH AND BEYOND
ENVIRONMENT
BIORHYTHM

BIRTHING******* DEATH

LIFETIME LEVEL OF FUNCTION ESTABLISHED
X_______________________________________X

Birthing and beyond takes us back to the new paradigm in which the birthing and pre-birthing processes are recognised as probably the ***key factor*** in establishing the ***level of functionality*** at which the organism will perform over a lifetime. It also includes the crucial ***intrinsic nutritional*** factor.

Environment includes such areas as nutrition (extrinsic), emotional/mental/cultural conditioning, suppression of acute disease phenomena (Drugs, vaccination etc), soil/ water chemicalization etc.

Biorhythm would include the normal rhythms of life and living, including exacerbations and remissions. It would, particularly, take into account the basic level of functionality of each individual.

Arguably, there is a genetic factor – possibly the homeopathic principle of taints or miasms. If this exists it may prove to be the early recognition of medicine's current toy, gene therapy, which we are now promised will lead to forecasts of our future health patterns and, in some cases, predictions of the likelihood of particular diseases such as cancer and coronary disease.

Interestingly, this will take medicine for the first time onto a ***horizontal*** assessment of health levels - other than the current crude instrument of family history. My own view, and it is only that, is that genetic patterns, tendencies, miasms or whatever other name is used, arise from a combination of influences. Most notable will be the ***environmental*** one and especially the ***nutritional*** issue, and more especially the

intrinsic nutritional one, all of which compound over many generations.

While the vertical assessment will always have a place in the healthcare field, there is good reason to believe that current practice is overly reliant on this methodology and that it is commonly capable of misinterpretation. The hitherto unrecognised ***horizontal assessment***, which is at the core of the ***predisposing causation*** processes in ***Bio Craniopathic*** philosophy, will henceforth assume not only a recognition in its own right, but will be seen to be the virtually always required component, irrespective of the symptomatology, or whatever other protocols may be deemed desirable, or necessary, for the resolution of illnesses.

There will also be a continuing inter play between these two influences over our lifetimes. For example, if we consider a theoretical comparison between two patients with, say, exactly the same level of functionality on the *Horizontal* scale (not possible I know, but please indulge me) - and all other things being equal - but one of whom followed a wholesome nutritional regime and the other not, the probability is that the latter would be subject to health breakdown more readily than the former.

Hence we arrive at the somewhat simplistic formula:

Predisposing (Master System functionality) + Precipitating (Lifestyle etc) = Level of Wellbeing

In this scenario the role of the hitherto unrecognised *Master System* is of paramount importance.

Chapter 16.

The Lifespan

I look to the future because that's where I'm going to spend the rest of my life.
George Burns

Among the more highly rated quests on Mankind's shopping list is that of the search for *eternal youth*, along with that of extending the lifespan of the species. The two are closely related, of course.

With all species there has to be a finite limit to which the lifespan can extend, and beyond which it becomes physiologically impossible to continue life. For example, the average lifespan of a dog is somewhere in the 10 – 12 years range and, however much we may wish for Rover to live forever, that just cannot happen. Even the more modest aspiration of, say, 20 years is not going to happen either.

The average lifespan varies enormously according to the species and, although this will vary over time spans – decades, centuries, millennia and beyond – we are ultimately limited by our physiological programming, the core design, if you like.

Within the essential characteristics of our own species there will be a host of variables. As I write top of the league table for longevity are the inhabitants of the Japanese island of Okinawa where they have more people over 100 years old, pro rata to the population, than anywhere else in the world. Japan itself occupies first place in the United Nations league table for longevity with an average age of 82.6 years (male and female), against a world average of 67.2 years and contrasted, in turn with, say, South Africa at 49.3 years – not even the lowest. There are many theories on the ageing process. Some are abundantly obvious as, in the case of South Africa cited above, HIV/AIDS is endemic in the country. Such a presence will clearly affect the longevity statistics.

Among the major theories of ageing can be found that of *Telomere Shortening* which looks at the effects of cell division over a period of time. Then there is the inevitable theory that "it's all in your genes", in which the view is that there is a strong inheritance factor. The excess sugar theory suggest that we reduce our intake of the stuff, thereby reducing the bonding of protein molecules together. The dietary theory generally, including excess fats intake (cholesterol), excess salt intake and a range of other, often differing opinions ranks high on the causative lists of ageing. Some hold that the endocrine (hormonal) function plays a major part. Nor can we exclude economic factors, the stresses in society, cultural influences, ethnicity, welfare systems and climatic input, among others.

There is certainly a general perception that we are living longer, a perception that is borne out by some of the available statistics (dislike that word). For example, in the United States, in 1930, life expectancy *at birth* was 60. By 2001, the average U.S. life expectancy *at birth* was 77. In apparent contradiction to that, according to numbers compiled at the University of Virginia, in 1830 there were 2,600 centenarians out of 12,866,020 people, or 2.02% of the total population. Whereas US census data indicates that in 1990, there were an estimated 37,306 centenarians out of 248,709,873, or 1.5% of the total population.

There is not necessarily agreement among the academic community that life expectancy rates are set to continue their upward expansion. At Cass Business School Wyatt Watson lectures in 2005, there were two lectures suggesting different conclusions. Professor James Vaupel, from the Max Planck Institute for Demographic Research in Rockstock, Germany, argued that life expectancy at birth and at sixty-five is likely to continue rising by roughly one year every four years. On the other hand Professor Jay Olshansky, from the University of Illinois, argued that life expectancy in developed countries will soon level off, suggesting that rising obesity levels in the United States would result in driving down life expectancy

In all, the subject is an extremely complex one. The available data on durations of life expectancy, including forecasts, is necessarily related to the *quantity* of life spans. The numbers of years. And we know that there are a vast number of factors which can, and will, impinge upon those figures, even within a given country, a given city or even a given household.

Nutritional variations are a pretty obvious influence on all our lives and, therefore, our potential longevity. So, too, would be the cigarette habit. Yet, hands up, we mostly know of those who defy gravity in these areas. There are those who defy all the rules about maintaining health, are at the extreme end of the "don'ts" and who do better than some strict adherents of the "do's".

So, the search goes on for the *magic bullet*.

But have we already reached the limit of our lifespan potentials, even in the more advanced societies? Or, are we close to it?

Chapter 17.

The Quality of Life

The secret of staying young is to live honestly, eat slowly, and lie about your age.
Lucille Ball

So much for *quantity.* Lurking in the background of any discussion on longevity, in addition to matters such as forecasting trends in relation to the *quantity* of life, is the equally, if not, more difficult one of determining the *quality* of life for each of us and the extent to which *quantity* and *quality* are inter-related in making life worthwhile.

The care of the elderly in Western society is increasingly *a concern*, both for those approaching, and into, their senior years, and for their nearest and dearest loved ones. It is probably no exaggeration to say that there is an increasing epidemic of *concern* on this one issue, raising a range of moral, ethical, financial and religious issues. At what stage does life become valueless, or even intolerable, for the individual?

As I write there has been a well-publicised case of a husband and wife jointly taking part in assisted suicide. She was 75 and suffering from terminal cancer. He was a famous conductor, 85 years old, partly deaf and almost blind. But he wasn't terminally ill. In both cases, however, the *quality* of life was markedly diminished.

In spite of advances, both medically and in society generally, most of us are aware of individuals and families facing either/or decisions of all kinds in relation to ageing issues. An increasingly common one nowadays is that of the dementia sufferer wherein the patient becomes progressively divorced from the surroundings. Along with this come the inabilities to perform the many personal tasks we all take for granted. And so it goes on and it is not my intention to moralise on any of these scenarios. We are all aware of their existence and of the fear that so often accompanies even the anticipation of the onset of any of these age-related changes.

All of which has increasingly caused me to ponder what improvements in the *level of function*, within the understandings of ***Bio Craniopathy***, might be brought to bear on this vexed question. If it is possible to superimpose another layer of enhancement on the totality of the body's *inherent functional mechanism*, then what might we expect? Even within whatever final limitations there have to be, imposed by the core design of the species and even without any changes to any of the other forces which play a part in determining our longevity – nutrition, culture, inheritance, lifestyle and so on?

One first has to acknowledge that, however much there have been, and will probably continue to be at least for a time, changes in the expectation of the life spans of all of us, these have been brought about to date mostly by a range of measures such as improved public sanitation, medical improvements, better nutrition and the host of issues, some already alluded to. But are we near to the plateau of these? Who knows, but, whatever further changes there may be from any of these sources, there must inevitably be a finite span of years beyond which it will be impossible to go, save the discovery of some Frankenstein substance or procedure.

This is a personal opinion, of course. The *design of the species*, of all species, will permit only that. In the light of this I want to discuss a theory which *might* allow for some painless and optimistic improvements in the areas of both *quality* and *quantity* of the human life span and which factors in the hitherto unknown body's ***Master System***. This is an entirely theoretical discussion, the value of which, if at all, will be unknown for many years ahead.

If we remove from the equation all those external forces and influences – lifestyle, nutrition, etc, etc – and pretend they didn't even exist, and strip down the length of our sojourn on this planet as being dependent solely on the activity of the *functional unit*, there will still be an *ageing process* at the end of which we pass on. That is the design and nature of the species. It may allow for the average life span to move to 100 years, 110, 120, even 130 years but it will be finite at some figure, just as that of the beaver is around 19 years, the chimpanzee around 40 years, the Galapagos land tortoise 193 years.

Within that span there will be a *process* of change from the beginning – birth – through to the end - death. In our own species, at the core of that process there must be a consideration of the *mechanism* which is central to the running of the process. Not the composition of the mechanism; not how we are put together. That is unalterable. The body's structures that are dependent upon that mechanism – the engine - our kidneys, for example, are different from those of a reindeer; and from a tortoise; and from a zebra. So are all the other organs and systems, all of which is to state the obvious. We are a *unique* human species.

What follows, therefore, is a modest attempt to suggest what might be the basis of some of the strands which determine the life processes and, as you might expect, are predicated upon the existence of the Primary Respiratory Mechanism's unique feature – ***movement*** - and my conviction of its essential role as the *engine of the life processes.*

At birth we will all be functioning at the highest possible level *for each of us.* In spite of whatever other weaknesses there may be incorporated into that level of function – and there will be some in all of us, as we know from the birthing traumas – the life processes will have been initiated and, at that stage, usually with little evidence of dysfunction. Symptoms, in other words, our usual measure of illness or disorder.

From Day 1 we are dysfunctioning, insofar as the ***Master System*** is concerned. If this is the ***Master System*** upon which *all* of the other systems depend and, irrespective of *any* other influences brought to bear on them, they will also be functioning *below par.* The descent into final dysfunction has already begun. And we're only a day old. The journey through life is ahead of us.

That inability to function at level 10 on our Richter scale will have begun the (usually) slow, but steady process whereby the body's inability to cope with the *burdens* imposed upon various structures, organs and systems becomes increasingly challenged. We recognise this daily around us. Symptomatically we might see the sequence as:

Asthma at 3 years
Tonsillitis at 10
Acne at 16
Knee "injury" from football at 24
Back "injury" at 38. Surgery
Prostate at 58
Ventricular tachycardia (fast heart rate) at 66

These events are milestones, or markers, easily identified as dysfunction but, in reality, are no more than peaks of an encroaching and developing *burden* within the system. What then has been going on over the years? We usually shrug it off with the all-encompassing explanation, "It's the ageing process". But what is happening from day to day, month to month and year to year? The answer is no doubt many things but I believe there is one very important component omitted in this explanation.

I believe that a major *effect* of the dysfunctioning ***Master System***, with its resultant impact on the other systems, is to progressively create what might best be called a reservoir of *baggage* within each of us. This is a *burden* which continues to build, layer upon layer, as the years pass by. The *burden* can consist of many strands such as mineralisation changes, often subtle, in tissue and cellular structures. There may be losses of elasticity of tissue; perhaps unnatural build-up of fats; maybe irregular fluid retention in cells or structures; perhaps abnormal levels of hypertonicity (tension) of tissue. What I am suggesting is entirely theoretical and the potential for the nature of the *burden* I have suggested is great.

But there is a two-way street here. The developing and expanding *burden* within the organism, whatever its form and nature, will inevitably and progressively exert a reverse *drag effect* back to the ***Master System***. It's as if the developing *weight* at the end of the ***Master System*** – anywhere in the body - begins then to add an extra *burden* to efficient ***movement*** which is, of course, the driving force behind the life processes.

It's as if when a small shunting railway engine, when hitched to a railway carriage, performs the task efficiently. And, there is little wear and tear back onto the engine. But, if it is connected to the increased burden of a dozen inter-city carriages, not only does its *functionality* diminish, but the *burden* of the task has the *reverse* effect of causing early failure of the engine itself.

There is a clearly defined *burden* when symptoms are present – asthma, diabetes, multiple sclerosis, etc – but the developing *burden* is present, is often subtle, particularly in the early stages, and continues to develop, whether symptoms are present or not. The reverse *drag* can have its origin in any, or all, locations in the body and will impact, among other areas, on the body's fascia.

The fascia is a tough sheet of connective tissue and which runs throughout the body from head to toe. Superficial fascia is fatty and lies beneath the skin. It forms a lining separating the skin from the deep fascia. Deep fascia usually encases muscles, blood vessels, organs and nerves; it also has a degree of elasticity. It's like the body's equivalent of cling-film, or plastic wrap, running through and around every tissue.

The fascia also becomes part of the covering of nerve sheaths – the epineurium – which, in turn, become an extension of the *dura mater*. Now, isn't that interesting? Here we have the *dura mater* effectively finding its way into every nook and cranny of the body. And, if there is some element of a *burden* along any of those pathways, the resultant *drag* created by that *burden* will finally find its way back to the *source* of the dural system – the cranium.

We can speculate that the increasing *burden*, from any area of the body, and imposed upon the dural *source* – the cranium - will then further decrease the motility of the ***Master System***. The amplitude of our *sine wave* will be impeded and will be increasingly laboured. The amplitude will diminish. The effect will, in turn, further result in a spiraling deterioration of the *burden.* Putting it another way the burden will increase, which means that overall health and wellness decreases. Over our lifetimes we are going around in ever decreasing circles in relation to the *level of overall function*. The greater the level of cranial *injury* from the outset, the greater – and speedier - will be the development and extent of the *burden*.

This, I believe, will be a very significant scenario in determining the life span of any of us. It will not be the only one and I make no claim to that effect. If we add to that some of the other abuses inflicted on ourselves, by ourselves, by others, by circumstances and so on, then we of course add to the *burden*. But the ever decreasing circle of *function*, from birth, and its effects on ***movement***, will surely be seen to be a prime, if not *the* prime determinant for each of us.

Which brings us back to the questions of *quantity* and *quality.* Even if there is currently a continuing trend to extending the life span, however miniscule, there is not necessarily a concomitant trend towards an improved *quality* of it. Perhaps for some but certainly not for all. It is not my intention to analyze any of the learned opinions in this area, save to say that we are all commonly confronted with observable instances of the elderly, and not-so-elderly, having little *quality* of life.

Indeed, it is commonplace to hear that on many acquaintances' wish list is that their preference is for a peaceful end to life, even if shorter, rather than an extended one with little or no *quality*. If my theory - and it is only that - is anywhere near correct, my belief is that both *quality* and *quantity* would be enhanced when, first, there is a recognition of the existence of the ***Master System***, and then we address the fundamental weakness in it, preferably pre-birth in the first instance and continuing throughout life. It will still be of enormous benefit, however, if that programme is not begun until any later stage in life. The only losers would be the pension providers. Time alone will tell.

Some will wonder that I have excluded the area of genetics from my discussion. It is a vast subject in its own right and I am no scientist. The debate as to the significance of our genetic inheritance pre-ordaining our lifetime health levels continues apace among researchers. Much was initially promised and from which there are already signs of retreat in some quarters.

My guess is, and it's only a guess, that the abnormality in genetic structure and which undoubtedly exists, and being related to particular "diseases", will prove to be an effect, rather than a cause. If so, the pursuit in this area for answers will prove to be a false dawn and another unjustified raising of hopes in those afflicted particularly, though not solely, with serious and severe illness. Time alone will tell.

In summary, the vicious circle may be portrayed something like this:

1. Birth >> lesioned *Master System* (MS)
2. Lesioned Master System >> commences *process* of establishing and building the *burden,* usually over many years

3. The *burden* >> further adds to the already struggling and dysfunctioning Master System – the "drag" effect
4. Further dysfunctioning of Master System >> additions to the *burden*
5. The *burden* >> further adds to the already dysfunctioning Master System – the "drag"

Until we arrive at zero movement of the Master System when all our worries are over.

Chapter 18.

Bio Craniopathic Methodology

Technology is very seductive, and it is certainly changing the way things are designed and made and taught. The problem is when technology has seduced you away from thinking about things as deeply as you should.
Arthur Ganson

The techniques that have been developed to change the status of the ***Master System*** to that of *anatomical flexion* took a number of years to develop and derive uniquely from the *philosophical principles* which underpin ***Bio Craniopathy***. There is only one objective - *anatomical flexion* - which addresses ALL systems simultaneously. That is to say, the whole person.

The methodology employed harnesses the alternating pressure changes taking place within the cranium to effectively decompress from the existing flawed (compressed) anatomical status of the patient's cranium. The TOTAL anatomy opens up, as should have occurred at birth. It is, literally, a physical re-birthing process, but not in any religious sense.

Technically, there are in total 29 bones in the human skull, including the hyoid (Adam's apple) and 3 in each ear, known as the ossicle groups. In practice, and for the sake of simplicity, I tend to exclude all of these when referring to the cranial bones and generally refer to the main body of 22 bones.

Central to the process is the relationship between the occipital and sphenoid bones which articulate at the *sphenobasilar synchondrosis/symphysis* (joint). The ***Bio Craniopathic*** technique directly engages the occipital bone in the process – referred to as the ***Bio Craniopathic Correction*** - along with the fibres of the trapezius muscle attachments to the squamous portion of that bone. By virtue of its articulation with the sphenoid bone any resultant action (or reaction) will be transmitted to the sphenoid.

The sphenoid, in turn, directly articulates with the following cranial bones:

Temporals (2)
Parietals (2)
Frontal (1)
Ethmoid (1)
Palatines (2)
Vomer (1)
Zygomas (cheek bones) (2)

Including the articulation with the occipital bone, the sphenoid then has *direct* articulations with 12 of the other 21 cranial bones. The 12 bones with which the sphenoid has direct articulations will, in turn have their own articulations with other cranial bones, giving the sphenoid *indirect* articulations with others. For example, the articulation between the ethmoid and inferior conchae (2).

The alternating pressure forces *within the head* – the Primary Respiratory Mechanism - and directed by the occipital are then received by the sphenoid which, in turn, is prompted to shift position, *anatomically*. That positional *switch* is then transmitted via the sphenoid's direct and indirect articulations to ALL other cranial structures, including the *dura mater*, so that, in total, they all take part in this waltz. It's a harmonious dance of follow-my-leader.

The ***Bio Craniopathic Correction*** – the **Procedure** - of the ***Master System*** is like pulling the trigger to release the latent stored up energy within the cranium. This was to use the body's own *intra cranial forces*. The recognition of the logic and need for this to happen is the unique finding of what is now known as the ***Bio Craniopathic System***. The next step was to determine the ***anatomical components*** required to bring it about.

And the final step was to develop these requirements into a methodology that was anatomically and physiologically sound, was logical, was efficient and was teachable. It was a re-booting of a mechanism that few even knew existed but which was at the core of all of the life processes.

The methodology also had to be one which leaves behind all notions of a *segmental* analysis – assessment/ diagnosis – and incorporated, at a stroke, a therapeutic application which addressed *all* cranial components *simultaneously*, including the ***dural membrane*** and, by extension, the spine itself. The organism's own inherent forces, and *intelligence*, are harnessed in a way that permits and facilitates the necessary *anatomical* disposition to take place.

The objective is one of *opening anatomy* in order to *free*, or *maximise, physiology*. And let's remember that physiology is merely function.

It is the reason why I believe the ***Master System(MS)*** reigns supreme, and is the one upon which all other systems are dependent for their functionality. After all, why only work on a patient *segmentally,* when for the most part that *localized* disorder is primarily being *locked in and held* from another source?

Chapter 19.

One Primary Cause

Every truth passes through three stages before it is recognized. In the first it is ridiculed, in the second it is opposed, in the third it is regarded as self-evident.
Arthur Schopenhauer

In earlier writings I expressed the recognition of the existence of the *lesioned* ***Master System*** as providing the underlying reason for generalised weaknesses, albeit often asymptomatic, throughout the body. I referred to this *lesioned* state as providing for a hitherto unrecognised ***predisposing cause*** behind a wide range of disorders. And that cause lay uniquely and only at the cranial level. In effect, the ***predisposing*** status itself was a state ***in which the anatomical status of the Master System was one of***

Overcontraction.

The requirement was therefore to change that to a status of anatomical

Relaxation.

The two words may sound somewhat strange in terms of anatomy. Yet, to me they encompassed a useful description of the targeted area – anatomy. If anatomy is *restricted, tensioned, misaligned, torqued, not open*, whatever other description is used, then it can usefully be described as ***contracted***.

It follows then that if the *release* of the *contracted* anatomical state will change the *anatomical contraction* status towards a state of *openness, unrestricted-ness, lack of restraint, freedom*, then the word *relaxation* seems as good as any to describe that status.

The freeing of anatomy is the essential pre-requisite to the maximizing of the Primary Respiratory Mechanism. Movement.

We are therefore ***anatomically contracted*** and therefore ***predisposed*** to the onset of a wide range of identifiable disorders mostly manifesting in *one or more of the body's traditional systems* – asthma, knee, skin, arthritis, uterine, gall bladder. The list is indeed long.

Functionally speaking, that ***predisposition*** arises *in the first instance* at the level of the ***Master System***. The symptoms may have arisen in any one or more of the other systems of the body but the underlying and ***predisposing cause*** will almost always have its origin in the ***Master System***

It is also important to note that:

Irrespective of symptoms, there ***is only ever one primary cause which is anatomical overcontraction of the Master System***

The physiological (and psychological?) effects of that overcontraction may result in ***either*** *over-relaxation* of tissue/structures **OR** *over-contraction*.

An example of *over-relaxed* tissue might be *aneurysm* or *varicosity.*

An example of *over-contracted* tissue might be *muscle spasm* (low back pain) or *atherosclerosis* (permitting plaque build up).

A few examples are worthy of consideration.

ASTHMA

The symptoms of asthma relate to a disorder of the ***respiratory system***. Most treatment programmes are aimed at the alleviation of the symptoms *in that dependent system* including the identifying of so-called *trigger* factors.

MENSTRUATION

Menstruation irregularities are commonplace among the female population and often the cause of much distress. Disorders in this area are deemed to be mainly within the remit of the ***endocrine/reproductive systems***. Treatment protocols are almost entirely directed to those *dependent* systems, including surgery without any awareness that these *systems* are themselves subservient to a ***Master System***.

LOW BACK PAIN

Perhaps one of the most common disorders encountered by most people in a lifetime, this disorder of the ***musculoskeletal system*** – more properly now the ***muscular system*** - is addressed by a plethora of protocols, ranging from acupuncture, manipulation, bed rest, medication through to surgery. All are directed to the *dependent* system itself and it is often a hope-for-the-best outcome by all concerned.

ANGINA

Angina pectoris is chest pain caused by lack of blood supply and oxygen to the heart muscle. We are therefore, symptomatically speaking, dealing with a disorder of the ***circulatory system***, another of the body's *dependent systems*, for which invariably treatment is directed directly to that system.

MULTIPLE SCLEROSIS (MS)

Here we have one of the relatively few disorders where the ***Master System*** itself is symptomatic. Nevertheless, since no such system exists in any field of medicine, it is generally attributed to a disorder of the ***nervous system***, which is itself an important *part* of the ***Master System***. MS is characterized by evidence of damage to *myelin*, a protective sheath which surrounds nerve fibres. Treatments are mainly drug based and symptom alleviating. Why does *myelin* become damaged? Is it related to cranial pump disturbance and its effect on cerebrospinal fluid (CFS) movement? Speculative, but a possibility.

The list of conditions is, of course, virtually endless. The foregoing examples are disorders which are well known and within our everyday understanding.

The ***Master System*** is *functionally independent* of ALL other systems in order to fulfil its role - ***movement***. Without all other systems, however, its existence and function would be without purpose.

All other *dependent systems* are without exception ***entirely and fully dependent*** on the ***Master System*** to fulfil their primary *functional* roles. None is an independent *compartment*, divorced from the others and there is the obvious inter-dependence between them. That dependency raises important questions.

If the level of functionality of the *dependent systems* is ***primarily*** dependent upon the level of functionality of the ***Master System***, how much more rational would it be to address the ***Master System*** IN THE FIRST INSTANCE for a large and wide range of disorders?

By doing so the body's inherent Life Forces are freed *from within* and the healing processes immediately set in motion. It then becomes illogical for therapeutic treatment plans to target the symptom area ***while continuing to leave in place the primary, or predisposing, causative processes***. These primary causative processes, if left untouched, will ***continue to impose their lesioned stress patterns on all other dependent systems.***

Such protocols have resulted in variable outcomes in our current healthcare cultures, some lifesaving of course, some temporary alleviation, some little value but, too often, followed perhaps months or years later, by the appearance of "another disorder", another name, another location in the body (commonly the laterality factor), and yet believed to be another unconnected illness. The practice is one of kicking the ball around the ball park rather than in to touch.

It is my fervent hope that those in the world of medicine and in whose fields some of the following disorders fall, will be willing and moved to investigate the potential benefits of the foregoing principles:

Kidney Failure with its attendant need for dialysis and transplants

Bone Marrow Transplants – the ***movement*** factor

Cardiac surgery – the *contraction* factor

Diabetes, Types 1 and 2 – left side *Master System*

Glaucoma – the possible connection between increased pressure changes in the eyes and intra cranial pressure changes

Obstetrics/Gynaecology – scarcely a female escapes disorders in this area. Early evidence suggests the ***Master System*** plays a major role in disorders such as endometriosis, dysmenorrhoea, prolapsus uteri and menorrhagia.

And others

Perhaps it's time to pause once again. By this time it will be appreciated that the ***Bio Craniopathic System (BCS)*** recognises firstly the *existence* of the ***Master System*** along with the primacy of that system in determining the functionality (including the essential health) of ALL other systems.

It follows that, *irrespective of the nature of a disorder or of the system involved (symptomatically), there becomes only one therapeutic objective:*

Change the status of the Master System to one of ANATOMICAL FLEXION.

In so doing *all other (dependent) systems are changed similarly and accordingly.* This should be the starting point (and often the finishing point) before attempting any other procedures or intervention at any secondary level. Severe injuries (depending on the definition of "severe") and life threatening situations, of course, are an obvious exception.

Chapter 20.

Segmentalism, Diagnosis and Opinion

Let Nature have her way; she understands her business better than we do
Michel de Montaigne

Current medical procedures and understandings have evolved over many thousands of years. Names such as Plato, Aristotle and Galen feature prominently in the annals of medicine, for example.

It would be a daunting task to do justice to the recorded history of even the more significant developments in such an evolutionary process spanning, as it has done, many of the world's great cultures. In the early Babylonian civilization (circa 4000 BC), centred in the areas of the rivers Euphrates and Tigris, there developed a system of medicine which included astrological movements as determinants in the diagnosis of disease. In the main priests were the physicians of the day and in the Babylonian tradition there was included a belief that the Sun was the source of all life and that the movements of the stars and planets had an influence in diagnosis.

The ancient school of Ayurvedic medicine had its origins in modern day India and is claimed to have its beginnings around 10,000 – 5,000 BC. Some claim that it is the oldest system of medicine known, and influenced the Chinese system and even the humoral system as expounded by Hippocrates in Greece. By any standards Ayurvedic medicine was very comprehensive and included among its tenets attention to diet and the use of herbs. The Ayurvedic system included fasting, massage, yoga and even steam therapy.

The Chinese system of medicine is both extensive and legendary. One of its important periods of development occurred *circa* 4000 – 1700 BC during which time the leaders were often chosen for their virtues of wisdom, leadership by example and good character. Notably much emphasis was placed upon living in harmony with Universal laws. The Father of Chinese medicine is claimed to be Shen Nong who, among many other things, is said to have identified hundreds of herbs to determine their medicinal qualities. Most medical systems throughout history included a number of modalities, often together comprising a comprehensive system. Chinese medicine had its origins in both philosophy and a spiritual dimension and were the basis of Taoism.

Perhaps the one common denominator in all the major historical traditions was the use of herbal remedies. Early Man, living much closer to the natural world than his modern equivalent today, utilized the plants around him for a wide range of purposes including food and clothing as well as for medicinal purposes.

Much of the accumulated knowledge of botanicals was handed down from generation to generation and in Europe during the Dark Ages were the main sources of medical care. In 1649 Nicholas Culpepper published his work, *A Physical Directory* and soon after he published the first herbal pharmacopeia for lay persons called *The English Physician.* Even today this work is still widely quoted.

The first *Pharmacopeia* in the United States was published in 1820. It contained an extensive range of medicinal herbs with listings of each herb's properties, usage and prescription levels.

The development of botanicals, particularly in the West, became increasingly sophisticated, evolving from beginnings which were at times astrologically linked through the empirical stages and to what were some profound writings such as those of the Physiomedical school, to which I have previously alluded.

Eventually, however, the pharmaceutical industry moved in to exploit this vast potential of healing properties. One of the early objectives was to determine which special property was contained in plants and which was the main *active ingredient*. This led to the practice of identifying, extracting and even producing synthetic equivalents of the active ingredients. All other ingredients of the plants, such as vitamins, minerals, oils, glycosides and alkaloids were excluded.

Physical healing modalities such as the use of herbs or conventional drugs, acupuncture, osteopathy, chiropractic have one feature in common and that is to *manipulate* the body's chemistry as the end product of the respective interventions.

Definition of *MANIPULATE* (www.merriam-webster.com) transitive verb

1. to treat or operate with or as if with the hands or by mechanical means especially in a skillful manner

2. to manage or utilize skillfully

All have their advantages and disadvantages and all have their criticisms of one another. Not least do they have their critics within their own groups.

The modalities themselves are mainly symptomatically driven even though most make claim to some degree of a wellness objective. That is, a state somewhere between a continuing absence of symptoms and a positive sense of wellness. There is an implied need to continue with a program of *manipulation* of the body's biochemistry, directly by medication (drugs, herbs, vitamins etc.) or indirectly by physical means (acupuncture, osteopathy, chiropractic) by ongoing protocols appropriate to that modality, if that sense of wellness or absence of symptoms is to be sustained.

For a considerable time now I have been conscious that, because our aspiration and expectation in healthcare is almost entirely symptomatically driven, the various schools of whatever disciplines, respond accordingly and the protocols of each are *addressed segmentally.*

By that I mean that the protocol becomes one of diagnosis relative to the symptom picture of the patient – rheumatoid, knee, skin, diabetes, MS, gall bladder, glaucoma, and so on. Symptomatic and local. Therefore *segmental.* The medical history of a patient may, or may not, be considered of some relevance but even when it does it is usually considered to have a segmental relevance. The symptoms are addressed and are generally not seen as a *part of a greater picture.*

For example, a patient diagnosed with atrial fibrillation (abnormal heart rate) and who had a history which included an episode of left shoulder adhesive capsulitis (frozen shoulder), would be considered to have experienced two separate and unconnected disorders. Each, in turn, would probably have been assessed, and addressed, *segmentally.*

This development is now well entrenched in the area of conventional medicine where specialism is the order of the day – rheumatologists, cardiologists, dermatologists, neurologists, oncologists and so on.

However, from whatever source a patient may seek professional help there arises a further difficulty which revolves around that professional's *opinion*. There is firstly the professional's *opinion* as to the nature of the disorder – the name – and which may be straightforward such as in, say, acne, but may also result in a patient being referred from one *specialist* to another. Even within the same specialties *opinions* may vary.

There is then the *opinion* as to the correct, or best, treatment plan and in this area *opinion* may vary widely *even within the same disciplines*. For example, for patient John what is the best drug for condition A? What is the appropriate dosage? Over what period of time? And for patient Elizabeth for the same disorder?

Then what other asymptomatic disorders are developing behind the scenes that no one knows about, least of all the patient, and which may influence that *opinion*, if it were known? To what extent is the amelioration (suppression) of one set of symptoms going to result in impetus being given to the onset of another new (?) symptom pattern emerging as a result of the prescribed programme? Such considerations will apply to most disciplines.

None of this is to deny that help in various forms, and degrees, is available for a wide range of disorders, and from a number of disciplines. Which is to say symptomatic relief and which is the main requirement for the majority of patients.

Mainstream medicine, if we exclude injuries and its attendant requirement for surgery, now places heavy reliance on the prescribing of drugs for a wide range of disorders. The drugs themselves originate from laboratory *manipulation* and are in no sense likely to be in harmony with the body's biochemistry. The objective, however, is simply to *manipulate* the body's biochemistry, often with powerful drugs, in order to relieve symptoms.

Herbal medicine by its very nature utilizes sanative drugs derived from Nature's bounty and is also intended to *manipulate* the body's biochemistry, usually relevant to a patient's symptom picture. The herbal medications generally have the merit of themselves being part of the natural order and being themselves free from laboratory manipulation. There is, however, a requirement for *opinion.*

Physical disciplines such as osteopathy and chiropractic are not generally thought of as being other than overtly *manipulative* of joints, ligaments, muscles, usually relative to injuries and such like. There is nevertheless an implicit objective of *manipulating* the body's biochemistry since so much of the body's systems function from neurological sources.

Definition

Chiropractic: *A system of diagnosis and treatment based on the concept that the nervous system coordinates all of the body's functions, and that disease results from a lack of normal nerve function.* www.medterms.com.

Similarly for osteopathy:

Definition

Osteopathy: A *system of therapy founded in the 19th century based on the concept that* ***the body can formulate its own remedies against*** *diseases when the body is in a normal structural relationship, has a normal environment and enjoys good nutrition.* www.medterms.com.

In both case the therapeutic determination and methodology will call for *opinion.*

As a modality acupuncture is generally thought of as being more in the area of *energetic medicine*. In a consensus statement issued by the National Institute of Health (NIH) there is included the following:

Findings from basic research have begun to elucidate the mechanisms of action of acupuncture, including the release of opioids and other peptides in the central nervous system and the periphery and changes in neuroendocrine function.

There is much debate within the acupuncture community, and between the differing schools, but this extract seems to point to the beginnings of a recognition of a *manipulation* of the body's biochemistry. Within that community *opinion* also counts for much.

In any, or all, of the alternative schools there was the pursuit of something approaching a comprehensive and conservative approach to healthcare. An obvious exception would be in the area of orthopaedics and surgery, although there may be questions as to the extent that surgical intervention is the best, or only, option at times. This was particularly true of the early pioneers in the fields of osteopathy and chiropractic but almost all have retreated from that aspiration.

The allopathic system of Western medicine now commands vast resources and is both commercially and politically dominant. It lacks any central philosophical base and its dominant theme continues to be symptom driven, *segmental*, with the chemical *manipulation* of the body's biochemistry, and therefore, *function* being the core tool. It's as if there is an on-going and constant trade-off between perceived benefit and none, too often one of trial and error - *opinion*. The attempt to *manipulate* one group of symptoms *segmentally* too often raises the suspicion that other structures in the body which are under stress, but are asymptomatic, are accelerated to becoming symptomatic.

To return to the theme with which this book began, the minute by minute, day by day, week by week *function* of the human body (and beyond) is not, and cannot be, a haphazard event. It cannot be disorganized. It cannot be without direction. It cannot be without purpose. It cannot be without intent.

The life processes which comprise each of us must be *intelligently* driven, and govern the *totality* of the relationships of *every single activity* going on at every level of our being. It is an intelligence beyond our conscious being and without which there would be chaos, which would simply constitute non-existence.

There must be a conductor of the orchestra. There must be a controller and, in this case, I have attempted to convey my own belief that, at the core of control and organization of every single activity is *involuntary movement.* I believe that until there is recognition of the existence of *movement* there will continue to be limitations to healthcare delivery.

The miracle of the potential for *organization, function, harmony, intelligence* already exists within each us. For reasons already discussed it is incompletely harnessed. Its origins are anatomical and its effects are physiological – function.

We are also comprised – physically at least – of the most incredible biochemical laboratory ever known. It is breathtakingly complex. Its analysis down to the zillions of microcosms that constitute the macrocosm that is each of us continues to be the pursuit of medical science in the apparent belief that, with enough energy and resources, all will be revealed.

If, however, we are prepared to concede that this magnificent organism that we call the human body is something more than a collection of parts, somehow or other apparently working together; that it is the most finely tuned orchestra, the sections of which themselves are miraculous, but which ***together*** function inter-dependently, harmoniously, intelligently and purposefully we can begin to see the emergence of a balanced ***whole*** which, in theory at least, requires no *opinion* or *manipulation* (by whatever means) of its parts (*segmentalism).*

Which brings us back to the ***Master System***. And there are probably two broad issues. Firstly, if the totality of function – physiology – of *all* of the body's systems originates from, and is determined primarily by, the ***Master System*** it will follow that just about every process including the myriad of biochemical ones, will be impacted accordingly. The degree of inter action and inter dependence between all of the secondary systems – respiratory, cardiac, endocrine, gastro intestinal etc.- will always be traceable back to the source.

If the source, the ***Master System***, is itself dysfunctioning, so then will that degree of dysfunction be seen in the other systems at a *predisposing* level in those systems. Such, for example, will its effects be manifested at the biochemical level of the body's function. To correct the dysfunctioning ***Master System*** will therefore result in the *automatic* correction of the perceived weaknesses in the secondary systems, not least at the biochemical level.

And *opinion* is eliminated. The body knows best.

Secondly, the limitations of the *segmental* application to Mankind's disorders will now be understood, however much such an approach may have been helpful to a patient. The *segmental* approach to most disorders is almost always symptom driven and excludes from consideration any *predisposing* element. This also applies to a high proportion of injuries in which the injury is a response to an asymptomatic, but *predisposing,* weakness in the first instance. On the highest level in the world of sport it is a regular occurrence to hear of household names of sports personalities with recurring or unresolved injuries and of the *segmental* programmes to which they have been subjected, including surgery.

In the graphic shown below it will be seen how the *functionality* of every system in the body is dependent upon the *functionality* of the ***Master System***. The basic weaknesses of the ***Master System*** will then be visited upon the dependent systems, in varying degrees, and which in turn, will have their *predispositions* to disorder largely determined by the status of the ***Master System***, but also influenced by the impact of life or lifestyle's *precipitating* influences and incidents.

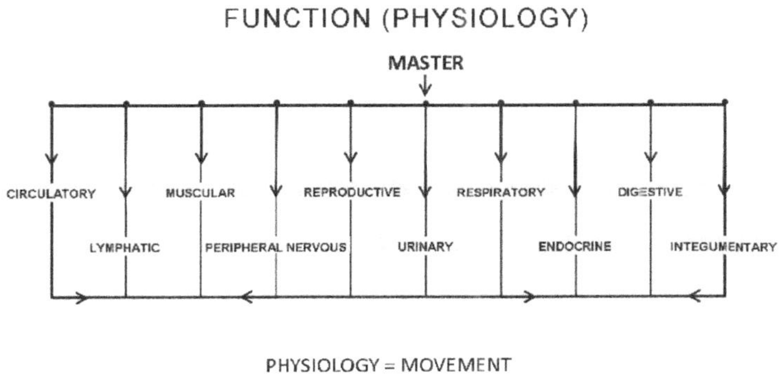

Fig. 10

If, therefore, a person becomes symptomatic in any of the above systems, it will almost always be *primarily* due to the presence of the *predisposing* input underpinning that disorder, and which will have its origin at the level of the ***Master System***. To address that symptom picture *segmentally* only is to omit the cause behind the cause and to leave intact the fundamental weakness continuing to feed into the secondary systems.

It therefore becomes an imperative, *in the first instance,* to recognize that, irrespective of the nature of symptoms and their location in whatever secondary system group, the status of the ***Master System*** must be addressed.. This is not to deny that other adjuncts may be useful, in addition, such as nutritional changes, massage, herbs and so on. But by changing the status of the ***Master System*** to a very specific *openness* the Bio Craniopathic practitioner is removing much *opinion* as to determining a therapeutic programme for a patient, and not least of all, a *segmental* one with its attendant shortcomings and even risks.

The body's innate *intelligence, purpose, organizational capacity* – the vitalistic principle – will do what it was designed to do, if released from its straightjacket of limitation of function of the ***Master System***.

And all this, *irrespective of the nature of the illness or disorder.*

None of the foregoing will apply in certain disorders. Most obviously, for example, in the area of serious or severe injury will there always be a requirement for "segmental" intervention, although it must be said that a range of lesser "injuries" require little more than Bio Craniopathic intervention – the *predisposing* factor.

Nor would it be possible to reverse genetically determined disorders such as spina bifida or Down's syndrome although there is no reason why such patients cannot be helped in other ways by the use of ***Bio Craniopathy***.

And, although changes in the status of the digestive system, for example, will enhance the ability of this system to function, including its ability to *assimilate, elaborate and distribute* nutrition from the food chain – ***the intrinsic nutrition factor*** – it will also profitable, particularly in certain disorders, to consider general nutritional and lifestyle matters.

Chapter 21.

Paediatrics

We've had bad luck with our kids -- they've all grown up.
Christopher Morley

The role of cranial dysfunction in children's disorders has been noted by earlier researchers. For example, Dr John E Upledger reports:

There exists a positive relationship between cranial motion restrictions and learning by disabled children, as well as children with a history of an obstetrically complicated delivery

There are, of course, a number of factors which may play a part in the causative processes. Some are controversial such as the MMR vaccination. Others such as nutritional status and genetic inheritance have been suggested but, however much such factors may, or may not, be a consideration, my own opinion – and it can only be that – is that they are largely peripheral to the issue. Their impact mainly results ***from the already weakened system*** being unable to deal with the secondary impact from these external forces, whatever they may be.

The term 'neurodevelopmental disorder' has become a term to describe major impairments such as the cerebral palsies

(CP) and embraces overlapping problems with speech and language, motor-perceptive function, behaviour, and learning.

Among these perceived intractable disorders is the autistic one with its "triad of impairments of social interaction, communication and imagination and a narrow, repetitive pattern of activities"(Wing, 1981; 1991). The incidence of the disorder is apparently difficult to estimate, not least because the diagnosis itself is challenged by the non-specific nature of the autism spectrum.

The cause, or causes, of the disorder continue to be researched and:

It is evident from research that autism can be caused by a variety of conditions which affect brain development and which occur before, during or after birth." (The National Autistic Society).

"Brain development"? Isn't that a major component of our ***Master* System**? However, all is not necessarily negative in those deemed to suffer from autism spectrum disorders (ASD). Michael Fitzgerald, Professor of Psychiatry at Trinity College, Dublin, Ireland, has argued that ASD characteristics are the same as those associated with creative genius. Among those whom he cited to have ASD characteristics is Isaac Newton who was recorded as having worked non-stop for three days without recognising day or night and often forgetting to eat.

Other famous names cited by Fitzgerald as having shown signs of ASD are H G Wells, George Orwell, Ludwig Wittgenstein, Mozart and Beethoven.

Professor Allan Snyder, director of the centre for the mind at the University of Sydney, said: *Autism ranges from the classical picture of severe mental impairment at one end of the spectrum to Nobel prize-winning genius at the other. Both extremes have core autistic features, such as preoccupation with detail, obsessional interests and difficulties in understanding other people's perspectives.*

The characteristic of genius often manifests in the area of music, mathematics and exceptional memories. It is as if, other than in those with severe mental impairment, all of the areas of *imperfect function* had been compensated by *concentrated function* into other areas, amounting to what we perceive as genius, or exceptional creativity, in those areas. As if the *underlying, but impaired, normality* had been swept into this other *normal* compartment as part of a *compensatory* mechanism, leading to identifiable, but lop-sided characteristics and behaviour. Indeed, are we all autistic in some degree but only a minority *clinically* so?

Similarly, and as an aside, are we all dyslexic but only a minority *clinically* so? I believe so.

My own experience in practice has been that at least the majority of my autistic patients were involved in significant birth, or pre-birth trauma. We can therefore only speculate on the possible neurological dysfunction that results from the birthing experience. Mediation from a ***Bio Craniopathic*** perspective has proved to be promising and offers significant help to these children – but with one major proviso. The nature of the ***Bio Craniopathic*** approach requires that the patient 'co-operates' with the practitioner. Which, for practical purposes, means that the child lies relatively still on a treatment table for, perhaps, two or three minutes without pulling away, pushing hands away and so on. If, however, the child is reasonably co-operative, then results can be very gratifying. In this respect, a suggestion from my colleague, Dr Vernon Rowe, may be helpful:

One thing that I have learned to do is to sit next to the child and gently stroke their knee or have mom rub their feet. Talk quietly while explaining what you are about to do. It is very important not to look at them, but continue to talk softly.

Then have them lay down while mom continues to rub their feet or legs.

Chapter 22.

Interesting Case Histories

For every failure, there's an alternative course of action. You just have to find it. When you come to a roadblock, take a detour.
Mary Kay Ash

This chapter was not originally planned for inclusion in the book. In the course of one of my many discussions with colleagues it was suggested I put together a chapter which might be called my "One Hit Wonders".

There follows a few of some of the more memorable cases that stick in my mind from many years in practice, 27 of them using the *Bio Craniopathic System.* My hope is that you find them interesting, perhaps even humorous.

Leukaemia

One of the very early, and dramatic, cases concerned a leukaemia patient. Let's call her Freda. This was quite early on in the days of the development of the *Bio Craniopathic System* and began with a phone call from the daughter of the patient. The daughter was herself already a patient of mine.

Her story was that her mother was suffering from leukaemia, had been through a series of unsuccessful medical treatments and was currently in hospital. The family had been told that the prognosis was negative and that she had no more than about two weeks' life expectation.

Could I do anything? To which the answer was that I had no idea.

I had no status in that hospital and there followed a lengthy discussion from which it emerged that the family had already discussed among themselves the options available – which were few – and had decided that they were prepared to sign their mother out of hospital and bring her to my clinic.

At the time I had a small and modest residential clinic but it was not geared for this level of illness, even though it ran 24/7. Eventually I agreed to see the patient at the clinic on the clear understanding that, if there was either continuing deterioration or, no rapid improvement, she would return to hospital. This was agreed.

That same day Freda arrived courtesy of the hospital ambulance, already attired in her night wear, accompanied by her daughter and ready to go. She was very ill. My recollection is that she had voluntarily stopped all medication and, on examination, she also had extensive skin lesions which were, in themselves, a source of considerable distress.

She was a wonderful lady and, as time was not on our side, we commenced a treatment programme immediately. In addition to the *Bio Craniopathic* treatment she was, like all other patients, put on an organic and whole food regime. That first treatment was late afternoon, as I recall, and I saw her first thing the following morning. And what a change!
I was shocked myself. The skin lesions had cleared by some 30%, the patient felt much better, she was stronger and was

able to walk around the rooms. Which she was far from being able to accomplish on arrival. I didn't expect this response and wondered if it was a fluke? Will this all fall back on us? Naturally, the family were thrilled but, like myself, feared that this might be perhaps the last kick?

To my own amazement, however, and that of the family, progress continued daily to the point where, even after a week, she was to all intents and purpose, a well woman. She was discharged after a total of two weeks and continued with follow up outpatient sessions for a number of months after.

But I was left with the question: if *Bio Craniopathy* can release the healing power to this extent, what other possibilities might there be?

The footnote to this tale is that I eventually lost contact with the lady and learned later that she lived a very full life for many years, eventually dying as a result of a fall from a horse.

Multiple Sclerosis

A lady presented with a diagnosis of Multiple Sclerosis (MS). Let's call her Maureen. She was in her early forties, was reasonably mobile and moved without walking aids. Her main symptoms were in the form of intermittent attacks during which time her mobility and balance were severely affected, as was her vision, all of which had called for early medical intervention. The overall deterioration from initial onset was slow but steady, and the prognosis was that she would inevitably become wheelchair bound.

We immediately commenced outpatient treatment, initially at approximately two weekly intervals and improvement was almost immediate. Her balance was much improved and her walking and energy were also markedly improved.

This programme continued for a few months until, on one visit, she announced she was pregnant. Gulp! I then realised I had not questioned her about family history and was unaware she did not have children. My next question was in the tentative form of, "How do you feel about that?" To which the answer was that she and her husband were thrilled, (hooray), even though this was a late pregnancy.

It then transpired that she had been unable to conceive and had accepted that there would never be any children. The lesson for me was to never omit to take a full family history. It was also reasonable to conclude that this patient's infertility had also been addressed through the changes brought about by the *Bio Craniopathic* programme and in addition to the changes in her MS status.

Infertility and MS – two for one. Not a bad deal.

Cancer

Here we have what was probably the weirdest experience I have ever encountered over all my years in practice.

I received a call at home one evening from my nurse to the effect that someone had left a young lady at the clinic to do what we could to help her. Could I come over right away? She was probably in her early twenties and on arrival I was informed that she had been dropped off – yes, dropped off – by a priest, who had offered no explanation as to who she was, where she lived, where she had come from, other than to say she had a cancer of the bowel. All we had was a first name – call her Liz. The priest had left without leaving any contact information and had gone long before I arrived.

The patient herself was clearly very ill and, on examination, had a rough and ready bandage and dressing around her abdomen which, when removed, revealed an open wound which was discharging putrid matter. Liz was uncommunicative and we could elicit nothing of the history but she was adamant she was not going to any hospital. Our guess was that she had already been in hospital care and had discharged herself.

What to do? This was not my territory. It was by this time late evening. The patient was in agony and we decided that we would at least offer her a bed for the night. We cleaned up the discharging wound as best as possible and I offered a *Bio Craniopathic* treatment. Frankly, I doubt if she really heard, or understood me, but, knowing that it would do no harm and, possibly, some good, I treated her before I left with the strict instruction to staff to call me if necessary.

Next morning I couldn't believe my eyes. The pain level had dropped considerably and the discharge had ceased! Liz was able to talk, although we could not get any more information about her or the circumstances surrounding the whole bizarre affair. Over the next week or so Liz made incredible progress and the wound closed up, with the pain clearing completely.

And then........One night Liz disappeared of her own volition. No one saw her go. No fee was paid by anyone. But we assume her health continued to improve. Was it a cancer? I don't know. It surely looked like it could have been but I'm no expert in that field.

It sounds like a story from a fiction novel, doesn't it? Well, it happened.

Diabetes

At my training seminars for practitioners we set aside a segment of time at which we call for case histories from the attendees. These are abbreviated summaries of significant health events, injuries and current health issues and from these are selected two or three cases for study. Each "model" is then assessed and is subjected to a variety of tests and challenges, which are then noted. Each "model" is then given a *Bio Craniopathic* treatment followed by checks using the same tests. Sort of pre and post tests.

At an early seminar, one of the chosen ones was a doctor who was Type 1 diabetic, insulin dependent. We'll call him Dr Tom. He had other challenges in addition. I don't recall the insulin programme he was on, or the levels of insulin intake, but before administering a *Bio Craniopathic* treatment it is necessary to be aware that in the event of an improvement of pancreatic function, there may be a need to reduce the insulin intake on the next shot, or shots. This is very important.

In fact, since it has been found that diabetes arises from the left side *Master System* lesion, it is equally important to be aware of the possible need to adjust medication with any diabetic patient, *even if the patient is attending for any left sided disorder – say a shoulder, a wrist, a left side sciatica and so on.*

With Dr Tom's agreement and in his full knowledge of what might be required, he was taken through a number of pre-checks, given his treatment and then post-checks. The latter indicated changes for the better. The following day all attendees were curious about Dr T and to the amazement of all present, we were given the report that Dr T had not needed, or taken, any insulin since the previous day. The same report was given the following, and last, day of the seminar.

The endocrine function of the pancreas comes within the orbit of the left side lesion and, I repeat therefore, that the application of *Bio Craniopathy* to *any* diabetic patient, irrespective of the disorder being addressed, contains the special precaution referred to above. This is not a contraindication to treatment, merely a special precaution.

Sports Injury

There are few sports that do not carry some risk of injury, varying according to the nature of the sport. Most of these will carry a heavy *predisposing* burden before the actual event which triggers the problem. It is usually the "event" that attracts the blame for the injury episode, rather than the underlying state of affairs – the *predisposing*.

One day I received a call from an officer of a local cricket club. For the benefit of American readers unfamiliar with this sport, cricket is the wooden bat and ball game played in open ground mainly in countries such as England, Australia, New Zealand, India, Pakistan, South Africa and others. It has some similarities to baseball. Most people in those countries know nothing about baseball, which is probably why they play cricket! Or, maybe it's the other way around!

The club officer's plea was on behalf of the captain of the team, a key player and the only professional on the amateur team. Let's call him Jack. It was a Friday and they had a crucial championship win-or-lose game on the Saturday. Jack had injured himself in the area of the right rib cage and was unable to bowl (pitch). He would also be unable to bat – that is, receive bowling from the opposing team. Bowling required an over arm action to deliver the ball, so this was mightily serious!

What could I do? Dare I let the club down with their big Saturday game? Just couldn't risk a lynching if the match was lost so off I sped late Friday evening to the clinic and there were Jack with the club officer waiting. Jack was a tall, wonderfully proportioned athlete, but was in pain even with little movement of the arm. Well, you've guessed it. He was immediately much freer and pain reduced after treatment.

The footnote is that the team won the game, won the championship and Jack reported that he had never bowled so well in his life. The lesson again is to address the real *predisposing* cause and not be distracted by apparent localised issues unnecessarily.

How often have I heard of the trials and tribulations of big name sports stars – and teams – wrestling with injury issues that I knew in my heart of hearts were resulting from *predisposing* structural problems. And wishing I could lay my hands on them.

Conclusion

How could drops of water know themselves to be a river? Yet the river flows on.
Antoine De Saint-Exupery

A re-evaluation of the current offerings on healthcare and the course along which it is being propelled, are long overdue. In the foregoing pages I've attempted to present a rationale which, however flawed, may open the way for a fresh discussion on the causative mechanisms of so much of Mankind's disorders. Not least about the need to examine the implications of all issues surrounding the birthing, and pre-birthing, processes.

Bio Craniopathy does not purport to make claim to being the all encompassing answer to Mankind's ills. But I believe it does offer a significant advance in both our theoretical knowledge of how we function – and therefore dys-function - and the practical application of that knowledge to the healing processes. It will be some time before the ramifications of any of the foregoing prove to be significant, not only in terms of health provision, but even in the wider fields such as sport, dentistry, crime, and even others such as the insurance industry.

We live in a world where the availability of information on any subject is there at the click of a mouse or the touch of a screen. Nowhere more so is this true than in the field of healthcare. The quest for answers grows exponentially and it is no longer enough to suggest, or imply, that those answers are often so technical that they are beyond comprehension by a lay person.

There has probably seldom been such an understanding, *in its simplicity,* of the essential *function* of each of us as that suggested by ***Bio Craniopathic*** philosophy. Of the *totality* which constitutes us. We continue therefore to be largely distracted from the obvious fact of our *self-healing* potential. I am cognisant that my suggestion of the existence of a ***Master System***, upon which all other systems are *dependent,* will challenge much present knowledge. I merely ask that it be given fair and impartial scrutiny.

At this time, the ranges of application of the ***Bio Craniopathic System*** have been found in practice to be extensive. Over a period of some 30 years it has continued to expand its knowledge base along with continuing refinements of its hands-on component. But I reiterate that we must never lose sight of the fact that what is commonly taken for a "local" disorder must *always* require that we address it from a *total* perspective. ***Globally***.

On the face of it, it will certainly seem odd, to say the least, to attempt to sort out the sciatic problem without even touching the patient's low back; or, of doing something about the skin problem by changing the cranial status only. Then, what about the cerebral palsy suffer? Or, the multiple sclerosis one? Or the angina one? Or the athlete's recurring ham string? The list goes on but, no matter what the commonality with any such conditions is, the people concerned are *dys*functional. ***Bio Craniopathy*** does *not* treat conditions or "diseases". This is important.

*The **Bio Craniopathic System** only treats the totality of a person.*

This is a very meaningful statement. It is exactly what it says and is a reminder of the need to move our thinking processes from a *fragmented,* or *segmental,* appreciation of disorder to a *holistic* one. The total person.

The aim is to open up the blocked channels to allow for the release of the damned-up flow, *centrifugally.* The aim is to *facilitate* the body to fulfil the mission for which it was pretty cleverly designed: that of achieving its maximum potential of *function,* and with all that implies – a level of wellbeing never before experienced and an unsurpassed resistance to external assault, be it in the sports arena, be it from stress, mental or physical, be it from the slip on the wet floor or, indeed from the "bugs in the air".

If the composite whole is at its highest level of *function,* if it is *co-ordinated* as never before, there can be the expectation that the journey through this life will be one of greater fulfillment and achievement, whether in the workplace, the family and home or the wider world.

Wellness is the key and the means of achieving that goal are *within us,* just begging to be released. An awakening to this simple truism is long overdue, but its absence is understandable due to any lack of awareness both of the existence of a *core mechanism* which drives every function taking place within us and which determines so much else. There is therefore the absence of any *obligation to ensure that mechanism operates at its highest level.*

It is quite illogical that, for the vast majority of disorders, the *primacy* of the body's innate healing potential is ignored. It ought to be the first port of call whereas it is for the most part discounted in practice. There are many reasons for this but chief among them, I believe, has to be the *absence of an incontrovertible and reasoned alternative to present day practice.*

Medical research, as presently generally understood, is a vast area of investigation and is itself often one of sub divisions, or compartments such as microbiology, virology, embryology and so on. One of the major fields of activity is in the area of pharmaceutical research which, in turn, is directed to the discovery of new pharmaceuticals (drugs), their development and evaluation, *almost entirely for particular diseases and illnesses.*

Hence, we have our cancer research industry, our high blood pressure medication, our statins for atherosclerosis. And so it goes on. We are now being managed to expect wonderful treatment for a range of disorders from the human genome project. All of which has evolved from the belief that the compartmentalized name of a disorder, or disease, is that which has to be targeted.

Whereas for most disorders the *primary cause* will be the localized manifestation of a basic dysfunction *at the source of the organism's total operation* which are then categorized and classified with a name relevant to the nature or location of the disorder. The symptoms.

However helpful the current approach to research has been in the pursuit of helping Mankind, there will continue to be a significant shortfall in the outcome until there is recognition that the driving force for all our functions – and therefore dysfunctions – originates from the ***Master System***.

To continue with the current fragmented, segmental, approach to addressing disorder is to perpetuate the presence of the underlying *primary* impaired interaction within the system and to continue to *predispose* the organism to further breakdown. This may be in the form of a recurrence of symptoms or to manifest as a “new”, and often apparently unrelated disorder.

The research industry, for that is much of what it is, must move on. It is in need of some philosophical reflection if we are to move on to a sounder platform of healthcare delivery, both in terms of costs and availability.

It is my fervent hope that ***Bio Craniopathy*** will light the way to a rational reconsideration of how we understand and deal with health and wellness matters. We must not be persuaded that the “secrets” to health lie only in the remote regions of what is sometimes euphemistically called “scientific” research some of which is, and has been, useful. Some of it not and some of it is even harmful.

If we refuse to be distracted by the often siren promises of the complex, the answers may well be found in the simple. Let us be always mindful that the organism *never wishes to be dysfunctional, was designed to be self-repairing* and *will repair if facilitated to do so.*

To do so we must, firstly and without fail, recognise the *existence* and the *primacy* of the body’s ***Master System*** over all other systems. The time has come to place the *conductor* of the great symphony orchestra, which is each of us, *on the rostrum.*

Appendix 1

A Tale of Two Truths

E Pur Si Muove
(And yet it moves – Galileo)

For many years there has continued to be controversy as to the existence, or otherwise, of an involuntary mechanism involving movement of the cranial bones, and other structures. There have been few scientific papers to support such a notion and, although there have been claims of palpatory findings of motion, these are largely considered to be too subjective to be of scientific evidence.

There also continues to be little commercial interest in this area. Research is expensive and is mainly funded and controlled by the pharmaceutical industry. Any outcome is therefore unlikely to satisfy their main objective. Even if very positive, it is more likely to challenge much of their *raison d'être* rather than assisting it. The same would apply to the plethora of often charitable organizations pledged to fund research in particular "diseases".

Which begs the question: is exploration in this area of cranial movement likely to be of significant value at all? Does it potentially hold promise of new understandings? Of a new dimension to addressing dysfunction in its many guises?

As the debate is set to rumble on, and even become emotional between some of the groups concerned, it is perhaps worth considering the core question: if there is *no movement* what, then would be the result? If *movement* is central to the life processes it seemed to me that there would be a resultant total absence of any life activity. Which would logically suggest an absence of the species. But that is a big "if".

The presence of our life forms along with all the life processes which are part of it, on the other hand suggest to me that there *must be an "engine"* supervising, directing, controlling and organizing every single life process that goes to provide function. Every engine has movement and, if such a mechanism underpins all of our myriad activities, it must be of the most incredible design. Which raise the further question: what then would be the origin of cranial motion?

Again, we are into speculation but I was impressed by the one suggested by Dr John Upledger on the possibility of an intra sutural stretch reflex mechanism, an alternating opening and closing of the sutures in a continuum. It shows considerable insight and has much to commend it. The application of the principles contained in this book are based on the premise that there is some form of mechanism as first suggested by Dr Sutherland. The practical outcome of that application would be null and void if intra cranial pressure changes did not exist. Which is not the case. The mechanism may, or may not, be as Sutherland suggested and time will no doubt reveal how close he was to perceiving both the nature of such an *involuntary mechanism* and its potential moment.

For this reason, I am personally content to leave behind the question of "proving" that there is movement of the cranial structures and move on to the question: how can there be living processes *in the absence of a moving mechanism present throughout life?* It is surely a truth yet to be acknowledged. One is reminded of a truth in another era and another context.

In the year 1633 it was the received wisdom of the day that the Sun moved around the Earth. Indeed it was the *required* wisdom. And so, when Galileo Galilei's discovery of the telescope in 1609 enabled him to confirm his beliefs in the Copernican system, that the Sun was at the center of the universe and that the Earth - rotating on an axis - orbited around the sun once a year, he immediately incurred the wrath of the Church.

Galileo was put on trial for his life before the Inquisition Court and given the choice between being burned alive at the stake or recanting his beliefs. The legend now goes that, as Galileo walked away from the Court, he was heard to mutter *sotto voce*:

"*E Pur Si Muove*" – "And yet it moves".

As Galileo's findings and declaration have proved to be true, so then it is suggested that Sutherland's findings will be held to be not only true, but highly relevant to the paradigm shift in healthcare that it promises.

"***E Pur Si Muove***" (in the cranial field)

Appendix 2

Training and References

Qualified professionals

Postgraduate training in the Philosophy, Art and Science of *Bio Craniopathy* is available and is vested under the authority of:

The Bio Cranial Institute International,
2601 S. Big Bend Blvd.
St. Louis, MO 63143
USA.
Toll Free: 888-738-7298.
www.biocranialinstitute.com

General enquiries

Please e-mail the Institute at: info@biocranialinstitute.com.

Patients

For a patient seeking reference to a qualified practitioner a current list will be found at www.biocranialinstitute.com/find-a-practitioner.

Note and Disclaimer

Bio Craniopathy is the result of ***original*** research developed over many years. A qualified *bone fide* ***Bio Craniopathic*** practitioner will carry the designation "CBC" (Certified Bio Craniopath) after his or her name. This can also be cross referenced on the above website. This information is given for the protection of patients as there are now individuals and organizations promoting incomplete and potentially harmful extracts of ***Bio Craniopathy*** *under other names.* We take no responsibility for any adverse consequences from their actions.

There are also other *bone fide*_cranial groups, mostly long established, whose principals and graduates operate with skill and integrity. An enquirer is therefore strongly advised to check credentials before committing to any course of action.

Made in the USA
Las Vegas, NV
29 June 2025

24225499R00115